COMMEMORATING LEADERSHIP IN HEALTHCARE

The New Jersey Hospital Association (NJHA) celebrates its 75th anniversary in 1993. Established as a seven-member association in 1918, NJHA now represents 112 acute care, psychiatric, long-term care, and rehabilitative institutions in the Garden State.

Through the combined efforts of its membership and staff, NJHA has become the focal point of the talents, energies, and resources for the state's healthcare provider community. Its mission: "To be the advocate for New Jersey hospitals, their systems, and the healthcare services they provide."

The New Jersey Hospital Association provides the leadership necessary to assist hospitals in planning, shaping policy, resolving controversy, and ultimately, improving access and quality of healthcare of all New Jerseyans. The core services—directed by the NJHA Board of Trustees—are advocacy and representation, political action, communications, issues management, and education.

NJHA's continued success in tackling the issues surrounding the organization, financing, and delivery of healthcare in New Jersey has earned it a reputation as one of the nation's premier hospital associations.

"Partners in Progress," Rod Hirsch

CELEBRATING INNOVATIVE LEADERSHIP IN HEALTHCARE

...Honoring the vision to serve the community and its people with commitment, compassion, and quality care.

Virginia Persing
Trish Krotowski

y-Law

...eld, N. J.

...orristown, N. J.

...mit, N. J.

nd Program

...an
...k, N. J.

...ERS
...ital, Elizabeth, N. J.

...KIS
...Hospital, Newark, N. J.

...ILLER
...ospital, Dover, N. J.

...MITH
...spital, Plainfield, N. J.

...A. HYDE
...tal, Jersey City, N. J.

...LLMAN, R. N.
...rial Hospital, Orange, N. J.

...H. MORROW
...solation Hospital, Oradell, N. J.

...S E. TALBOT
...City Hospital, Newark, N. J.

First Annual Meeting

OF THE

New Jersey Hospital Association

Office of the Chairman
116 Fairmount Avenue, Newark, N. J.

BOARD OF TRADE ROOMS
800 Broad Street, Newark, N. J.

Thursday, June Twenty-six, Nineteen-nineteen

CHARLES E. TALBOT, Temporary Chairman
Superintendent Newark City Hospital

I
n 1918 a quiet, unnoticed meeting occurred in Newark, New Jersey that would affect the course of healthcare in the United States. The small gathering of private citizens was far removed from the convenings of heads of state then negotiating a new world following the Great War. Yet, the meeting in New Jersey was nontheless auspicious and indicative of the era that was emerging. Seven hospital executives came together at Newark City Hospital and formed an organization—one of the first—to address the common concerns facing the state's rapidly growing and changing hospitals. Since then, for 75 years, the New Jersey Hospital Association (NJHA) has been a pacesetter, providing innovative leadership in healthcare in New Jersey, the nation, and the world.

The end of World War I in 1918 swept away forever the old, static order of monarchies ruling by absolute right and of social classes living according to preordained fate. Gone were all the fixed, centuries-old attitudes. The new view of the world, shaped in part by Einstein's theory of relativity and Freud's theory of the human unconscious, was one of change and complexity. It was a world that—while not necessarily "safe for democracy"—emphasized the rights and the power of the common man, fostering the ideals of the West's democracy and Russia's Bolshevik Revolution. Responsibility for the course of human events was in the hands of ordinary citizens who, collectively, could determine their own destinies.

COMING TOGETHER

The Founding of the New Jersey Hospital Association

New Jersey—the "In" State

The time, 1918, and the place, New Jersey, were ideal for the endeavor that was to influence the history of America's healthcare. New Jersey, highly urban and densely populated with a rich diversity of people, has been characterized since its beginning by three "ins": ingenuity, inventiveness, and innovation. New Jerseyans invented the first stagecoach (the "Jersey wagon"), steamboat, submarine, suspension bridge, locomotive, sewing machine, commercial plastic, electric light, motion picture, flexible photographic film, structural iron beam, commercial canning process, web printing press, rubber conveyor belt, alkaline battery, and transistor. Thomas A. Edison's most brilliant invention was probably the modern research laboratory itself, and ever since, New Jersey has been called the "research state."

New Jersey's penchant for ingenuity and innovation continued throughout the Industrial Age and into the Information Age, with its arenas of public affairs and human services. Perhaps because of its large, pluralistic population living in a diverse geographical area, New Jerseyans developed a genius for the political process and became skilled in debate, negotiation, and inclusion.

Also, perhaps because of its relatively small size and its proximity to New York and Philadelphia—Benjamin Franklin referred to New Jersey as "a barrel tapped at both ends"—New Jersey has always been an exporter of goods and ideas to the nation at large.

Innovation in Healthcare

In no other area has New Jersey's talent for innovation been more apparent than in healthcare. New Jersey was the first state in which humane treatment for the mentally ill, championed by Dorothea Dix, became public policy; the first state in which penicillin was used on human subjects; and the first state in which the antiseptic theories of Lister and Pasteur were adopted on a large scale, as the basis of the Johnson & Johnson first-aid products.

New Jersey has not only been a leader in science and technology, but in healthcare planning and policy, as well. In its 75 years of existence, the New Jersey Hospital Association has been responsible for a number of national "firsts," including:

- The first state hospital association library
- The first radio network linking hospitals
- The first hospital disaster drill
- The first program for visiting hospital executives from developing nations
- The first nationally recognized nurse refresher program
- The first licensed state hospital association insurance program
- The first statewide hospital group computer service
- The first statewide hospital engineering program
- The first statewide hospital energy conservation program
- The first hospital employee health coverage alternative to Blue Cross/Blue Shield
- The first statewide voluntary hospital budget review system
- The first payment plan to contain costs based on Diagnostic Related Groups, which became the basis for the national Medicare reimbursement program
- The first state Health Research and Educational Trust, formed as an affiliate corporation of NJHA, to develop a large number of nationally acclaimed public information programs
- The first state association to gather its affiliates and related healthcare organizations in one central location, on a large scale
- The first state association to include all of the state's hospitals in its membership, making the history of NJHA largely synonymous with the history of its hospitals

Each of these innovations was a creative—and usually proactive—response to the changing needs of healthcare and hospitals in each decade since the founding of NJHA.

Optimism and Expansion—the 1920s

NJHA was established in 1918 at a meeting of representatives from seven hospitals in northern New Jersey: Newark City Hospital, Muhlenberg Hospital in Plainfield, Elizabeth General Hospital, Hudson Tuberculosis Hospital and Sanitarium in Secaucus, Morristown Hospital, Paterson General Hospital, and Christ Hospital in Jersey City.

The agenda of the first annual meeting of NJHA in June 1919 illustrates the growing regulation and government involvement in healthcare, as well as an eagerness to share the common problems and experiences of hospitals. The morning session was a speech by the commissioner of New Jersey's Department of Institutions and Agencies (now the Department of Human Services) on "The New Commission for the Physically Handicapped in Relation to Hospitals"; an afternoon session featured a talk by a physician and former hospital administrator on "How I Met Some of My Problems." The constitution and bylaws adopted in 1919 state that the purposes of NJHA were "the study of hospital problems, standardization of methods in hospital management, promotion of proper legislation, the securing of uniform accounting."

Along with its national counterpart, the American Hospital Association, which came into being at the beginning of the 20th century, and the other fledgling state associations, NJHA was in the vanguard of the movement to create efficient, accredited hospitals that operated according to accepted scientific and professional standards. The early part of the 20th century was marked by advances in science and technology and also by controversy over physicians' credentials. Medical schools of questionable quality were closed and standards became more uniform and stringent.

NJHA met regularly through 1921 and 1922, and membership grew to include representatives from hospitals in the central and southern parts of the state, including Middlesex General Hospital in New Brunswick, Cooper Hospital in Camden, and the Atlantic County Tuberculosis Hospital. Because of the difficulty of transportation in the 1920s—the automobile was just coming into popular use—the association did not meet for a time. In 1924, however, interest was revived and the association met regularly, with an increasing number of representatives from hospitals statewide.

By the mid-1920s, NJHA was one of the strongest state hospital associations in the country and hosted the national convention of the American Hospital Association in Atlantic City in 1926 and 1929. While it grappled with increasingly complex issues, the association maintained a human warmth and scale. An "historical sketch" in the 1927 yearbook captures the tone of an early gathering: a roundtable meeting was held "at which the intricate hospital functions were discussed in a friendly and open manner by the entire membership."

*O*ne of the seven institutions that helped establish NJHA, Morristown Memorial Hospital boasted a fully equipped operating room in 1900.
Courtesy, Morristown Memorial Hospital

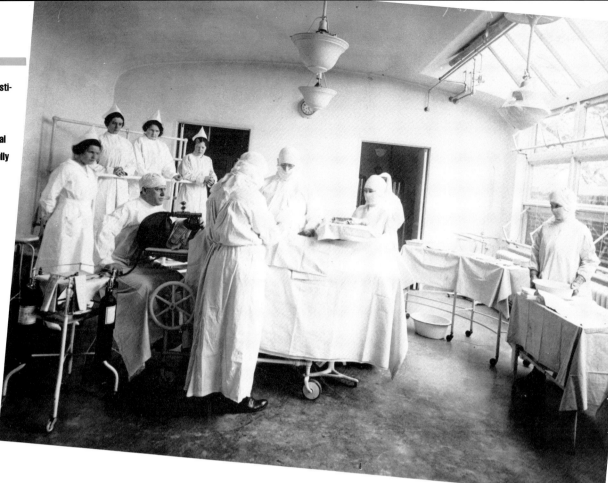

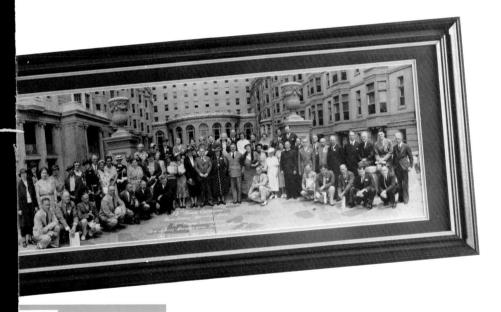

*N*JHA hosted the Atlantic City convention of the American Hospital Association in 1926 and 1929. New Jersey hospital programs and initiatives—such as the reception for foreign delegates in 1926—gained national attention.
Courtesy, New Jersey Hospital Association

*T*o address the shortage of qualified personnel, in the 1940s, NJHA recommended minimum salaries for nurses, like these 1948 graduates from Saint Michael's Medical Center in Newark.
Courtesy, Saint Michael's Medical Center Division/Cathedral Health Services, Inc.

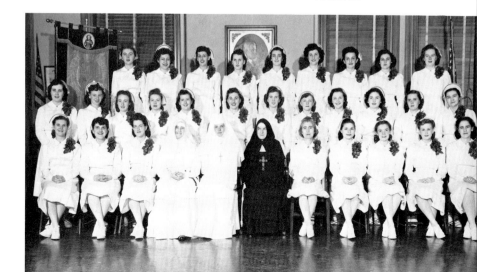

Hard Times and the New Deal—the 1930s

NJHA first proved its mettle during the hard years of the 1930s. The worldwide depression that began with the crash of the American stock market late in 1929 brought the economy to a standstill and resulted in the unemployment of 12 million people. Because of the suffering and hardship on such a massive scale, the federal government became directly involved, really for the first time, in the human welfare of its citizens. This was a radical shift for the United States. Its founding fathers had not seen this role as the business of government, and even the Depression President Herbert Hoover was opposed to government involvement "in the relief of individual suffering."

Franklin Roosevelt, however, offered the American people a New Deal of "relief, reform, and recovery." Congress passed the Social Security Act and initiated the Works Progress Administration (WPA), which put millions of Americans to work constructing roads, bridges, and buildings.

The entrance of the federal government into the realm of social welfare had far-reaching effects on the healthcare industry. In 1932, NJHA was instrumental in establishing the Hospital Service Plan of New Jersey (Blue Cross), with the cooperative effort of 17 New Jersey hospitals. Because New Jersey had taken an early initiative in this area, the autumn 1934 issue of the NJHA *Quarterly Bulletin*, covering that year's AHA convention in Philadelphia, reported, "Group hospitalization and federal aid, so well known to us in this state, were prominent in the program daily." A message from NJHA's chairman, William J. Ellis, in the same issue, indicated how the association proved itself in the 1930s: "High points of achievement include the enhancing of public confidence in hospital service and the enlistment of cooperative financial assistance for general hospitals from the New Jersey Emergency Relief Administration."

New Jersey's hospital "lien law," which provided hospitals adequate reimbursement for the care of "compensation" cases, was the first legislation of its kind and a model for federal legislation. In the winter 1934 issue of the *Quarterly Bulletin*, New Jersey Governor Harold G. Hoffman summarized: "The hospitals of New Jersey have furnished a brilliant example of effective service under difficulties of increasing need and accompanied by decreasing resources during the last five years. . . . New Jersey has been one of the states to recognize the merit of its healing services and to take the steps necessary to adequately uphold the hands of those charged with its work."

Triumph and Prosperity—the 1940s

During and after World War II the economy boomed; it was the war, not the New Deal, that ended the Great Depression. Still, during the 1940s—and to the present day—New Jersey hospitals continued to find ways to provide adequate healthcare to the indigent. In 1945, the NJHA Welfare Committee recommended that legal responsibilities for providing high-quality hospital care for those unable to pay be clearly defined and that the financial status of hospitals should not be jeopardized by rendering this care.

It was during the 1940s—because of medical advances resulting, at least in part, from the war—that the modern hospital was born. A major breakthrough was the development of sulfa drugs and penicillin to combat previously mortal diseases. Surgical procedures were more successful and became more sophisticated because of the reduced risk of infection.

With the influx of wounded solders returning from the battlefields, healthcare leaders addressed the inadequacy of the nation's hospital facilities. In 1946, Congress enacted the Hospital Survey and Construction Act, popularly known as the Hill-Burton program. This legislation was intended to stimulate local communities to renovate and build modern hospitals, based on need, according to population density. The expansion of the 1940s also sorely pressed the hospitals' manpower needs. The shortage of nurses, a cyclical problem that continues to the present time, first became an acute problem in this era. In response to this need, NJHA recommended minimum salaries for nurses.

NJHA was growing to keep pace with the rapidly expanding hospital system and healthcare industry. In 1947 the association hired J. Harold Johnston as its first full-time executive secretary, developed its first budget (of $12,035), and listed 57 New Jersey hospitals in its membership. A significant development was the formation of the Middle Atlantic Hospital Conference—now the Middle Atlantic Health Congress—by NJHA and its sister associations in New York, Pennsylvania, and Delaware.

Suburbs and Space Technology—the 1950s

In the 1950s, Americans retreated to the suburbs and advanced into space. Both movements had far-reaching effects on hospitals and healthcare. The flight of middle-class Americans to the suburbs left inner-city ghettos. City hospitals were faced with large numbers of indigent patients who suffered from the health problems associated with poverty.

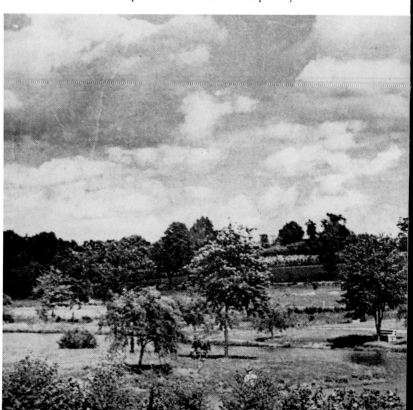

The "space race" was the impetus for technological advances that brought astounding breakthroughs in healthcare. During the 1950s the federal government began a massive investment in biomedical research through the National Institutes of Health. The increasing super-specialization and use of sophisticated equipment made hospitals, more than ever, the focal point of healthcare in America. American hospitals experienced enormous growth.

As a result, more—and more highly trained—medical personnel were needed. New Jersey was in the forefront of addressing the urgent manpower issues of the 1950s. NJHA revised New Jersey's Nursing Practice Act and advised the Board of Nursing on nursing school curricula. Also, at a time before unions were perceived as having the right to demand collective bargaining in hospitals, NJHA developed a series of institutes to explore labor-management relations and commissioned nationally recognized studies of labor relations in hospitals.

The Cold War—and the threat of a nuclear one—pervaded the 1950s. The National Fallout Shelter Program, developed by the American Hospital Association, was implemented in New Jersey. NJHA devised the first disaster emergency plans for hospitals and issued a manual, used nationally, on disaster planning. The challenges facing America's hospitals, however, were posed not by foreign aggression but by growing domestic issues and unrest.

Human Rights and Healthcare Planning—the 1960s

The 1960s can be understood as a decade in which the concept of human rights—so basic in the founding of the United States—was claimed by and extended to all citizens regardless of race, gender, social class, or ethnic background. The Great Society, an extension of the New Deal philosophy that government should be responsible for the welfare of its citizens, devised social programs of services to which Americans were entitled. Access to high-quality healthcare came to be seen as a basic right, not a charity dependent on the goodwill of others or a privilege based on one's ability to pay.

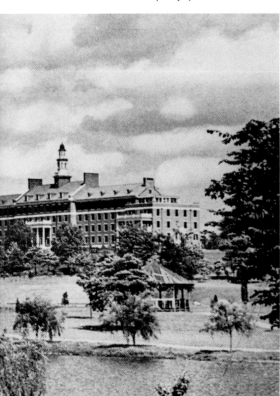

*R*oosevelt Hospital in Metuchen, New Jersey, was a WPA project, constructed—along with Roosevelt Park—in 1936.
Courtesy, Roosevelt Hospital

In the early years of the decade, NJHA was instrumental in implementing the Kerr-Mills program in New Jersey, which provided medical care for the indigent and low-income elderly. The association was also largely responsible for expanding, for the first time, health services and clinics to New Jersey's migrant farm workers. The landmark healthcare legislation of the decade, in fact of the half-century, was of course Medicaid, providing healthcare for the nation's "deserving" poor, and Medicare, ensuring healthcare for the nation's elderly.

The increased complexity and costs of healthcare added to the need for research and planning, and New Jersey was in the vanguard. NJHA developed the first state hospital association institute in regional planning, and the Regional Planning Council was started in 1963 under the auspices of NJHA. Under Jack W. Owen—one of the nation's most respected healthcare leaders, who served in the American Hospital Association (AHA) before becoming NJHA's second president—NJHA established the Health Research and Educational Trust (HRET). The purpose of HRET was to study issues, explore innovations in the healthcare field, and encourage new, imaginative courses of action. Many of New Jersey's healthcare "firsts"—such as the first hospital industrial engineering program, the first shared computer program, the first series of nationally used hospital training materials produced by a state association, and the first malpractice liability insurance program for member hospitals—were initiated in the 1960s by HRET. Also, a Nurse Refresher Program, which offered 100 courses, was attended by nearly 1,000 nurses, 65 percent of whom returned to practice.

The Concept of a Center—the 1970s

HRET continued to be responsible for New Jersey "firsts" in the 1970s, especially in the area of education and public awareness. New, first-of-their-kind programs included a health careers program; a mobile health education unit; an infant car seat public awareness campaign; a library; and Tel-Med, a program of recorded informational messages reached by calling a toll-free number. Building on the success of HRET, NJHA founded additional spin-off corporations in the 1970s. Each of these corporations—which have been added, reorganized, or eliminated over the years as needs changed—was established to enable NJHA to fulfill its mission: to be the advocate for New Jersey hospitals and the healthcare services they provide.

As the complexity of healthcare increased and new corporations were formed in addition to NJHA's councils and committees, the concept of a Center for Health Affairs (CHA) was born. The center, envisioned as a place where hospitals, organizations, and agencies could work together on issues, opened in 1977 on the growing Route 1 corridor in Princeton. It houses NJHA and affiliated corporations, as well as other health-related organizations. In addition to day-to-day sharing among the resident organizations, the center hosts more than 1,000 seminars, workshops, and conferences each year, attended by more than 30,000 people. A central resource for all healthcare providers in the state, the

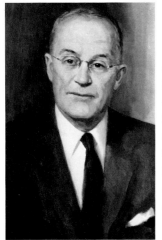

***B*y 1947, NJHA had grown large enough to hire J. Harold Johnston as its first full-time executive secretary—the equivalent of today's association president.**
Courtesy, New Jersey Hospital Association

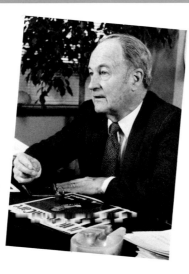

***J*ack W. Owen—NJHA's second president—expects many more challenges in his long-time career in healthcare. He says, "The problems of the hospitals in the '90s will require all the creativity we can muster."**
Courtesy, New Jersey Hospital Association

***N*JHA chairman William J. Ellis, in 1934, wrote: "Members of the New Jersey Hospital Association may, I believe, take genuine pride in the notable achievements which have been brought about on behalf of hospitals in the face of economic calamity national in scope."**
Courtesy, New Jersey Hospital Association

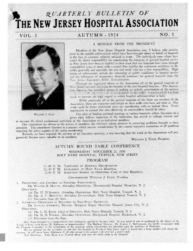

center maintains a centralized data base known as The Hospital Information System (THIS), another New Jersey "first." A group purchasing program administered at the center, which has saved New Jersey hospitals millions of dollars, has been a model for other state associations across the country.

Today, the Center for Health Affairs campus houses NJHA; NJHA Insurance Funds; the Health Research and Educational Trust of New Jersey; HealthPAC of New Jersey; CHA Inc. (offering administrative, data base, legal, travel, strategic planning, purchasing, human resources, marketing, conference and facility services, among others, through its Corporate Services Division); and CHA's divisions of Middle Atlantic Services (MASC) and Center for Health Affairs Insurance Services (CHAIS). The MASC division includes NJUP Plus, Group Purchasing, Advantage Pharmacy, Evergreen Financial, and group benefits administration. CHAIS consists of Princeton Claims Management; administration of the Healthcare Employees Federal Credit Union; and pension, tax-sheltered annuity and workers' compensation administration.

The restructuring of NJHA and its affiliates within the Center for Health Affairs—which has made possible so many imaginative programs and cooperative endeavors—was itself a major innovation. As hospitals observed the restructuring of the association, many saw the need for similar restructuring of their own organizations. Some New Jersey hospitals modeled their structures after the association and developed corporations for various purposes, to further their missions and to bring dollars back into patient-care delivery.

Containing Healthcare Costs—the 1980s

In no other way and in no other decade has New Jersey's healthcare system been so recognized as a national pacesetter than in the 1980s for applying Diagnostic Related Groups (DRGs) to a reimbursement model. The DRG reimbursement system, simply stated, classifies illnesses into nearly 1,000 categories, or diagnostic groups, for which a uniform price is set based on the average bill for patients with that type of illness. This original approach to curtailing escalating healthcare costs, implemented for all patients in New Jersey in 1980, became the model for the federal Medicare program.

The DRG system forced New Jersey hospitals to be even more efficient. In the 1980s, New Jersey's hospitals were cited by a national study as the nation's most cost effective, with the lowest charge for care of any state in the country. New Jersey hospital costs still rank among the nation's lowest and are strikingly lower than other states in the Northeast. Remarkably, this effort to contain costs was achieved without sacrificing the quality of healthcare and while pursuing new initiatives to address the nursing shortage, community outreach, and care of the elderly.

In many ways New Jersey, because it is the nation's most urban and densely populated state, is the first to confront problems that will soon, or eventually, face other states. Hospitals within large, aging cities, in order to meet the needs of their communities, have evolved into medical centers, providing ambulatory healthcare as well as a variety of health-related social services. Also, at a time when the nation's population is aging, New Jersey—with the second oldest median-aged population, after Florida—has been pointing the way in healthcare for this group. Home healthcare programs, geriatric clinics, day care centers for adults, and long-term care facilities located within or adjacent to hospitals are some of the notable initiatives in the state.

New Jersey can perhaps be proudest, however, of the fact that by law (Chapter 83) no one is ever turned away from its acute care hospitals for inability to pay. In 1987, unprecedented legislation, the Uncompensated Care Trust Fund Act, provided a new mechanism to guarantee access for indigent patients and a funding mechanism so that hospitals in low-income areas would not face financial insolvency for providing that care. Former New Jersey Health Commissioner Molly Joel Coye, M.D., commenting on the law, observed, "It is an exciting development and one which sends a message from New Jersey that much of the country is missing. With hospitals in other states turning uninsured patients away, New Jersey is demonstrating that it is possible to care for the poor and still contain hospital costs."

The Past as Prologue—the 1990s and Beyond

The nation's healthcare system—the world's most sophisticated and most costly—faces enormous challenges and changes in the 1990s. The American public, according to the media, the polls, and the political platforms it supports, perceives the healthcare system as in a state of crisis. According to Jack Owen, problems of affordability and access will be major concerns. "The 1990s are much like the 1960s, because accessibility is the problem," he says. "But in the '60s, it was the question of accessibility for the elderly and the poor. In the '90s, it's a matter of accessibility for the middle class." Healthcare leaders such as Owen, who says that "we've used up all the easy answers," feel that some kind of nationally mandated universal insurance coverage is inevitable. As for the role of New Jersey, since the states are the laboratory of the federal government, it is an opportunity for NJHA and its affiliates to explore solutions.

Early in 1990, NJHA published the *President's Task Force Report on Regulatory Change*, which made significant recommendations to deal with issues such as funding uncompensated care, and the management of health insurance providers. One of the specific recommendations of the report

was that there be some kind of minimum insurance coverage for all New Jerseyans. On the national level, NJHA is working with key legislators and with healthcare administrators in other states to identify issues and suggest approaches and methodologies.

Current NJHA President Louis P. Scibetta says New Jersey is looking at hospitals and healthcare "from as broad a perspective as possible" and feels that NJHA will make a difference in the future of the system. "The association provides the forum for the participants and it provides the leadership. Leadership is where the risk is, taking people in new directions and promoting change."

NJHA demonstrated continued leadership in helping to pass New Jersey's most significant healthcare reform legislation in more than a decade, designed to reform the hospital payment system. Key to behind-the-scenes reform negotiation, NJHA created a coalition of business, labor, insurance, and other representatives to suggest and analyze mutually acceptable elements of long- and short-term healthcare reform. The coalition's comprehensive proposals were presented to the governor in November 1992. By the close of the year, the Health Care Reform Act of 1992 was signed into law, dramatically changing the hospital payment system and the hospital operating environment. Among various provisions, the act provided payment for care of the indigent by diverting funds from the state's Unemployment Insurance Fund; created a payroll-tax trigger if the fund falls below a designated level; continued the current Hospital Rate Setting Commission for one year; eliminated DRG billing and enabled hospitals to bill actual charges individual patients incur; and provided a $100 million subsidy to hospitals with high Medicare populations. The law also created New Jersey SHIELD to subsidize health insurance for the working uninsured and temporarily unemployed. The most controversial provision set a hospital payment "revenue cap" based on historical factors.

At the beginning of 1993, NJHA was vigorously pursuing changes to the legislation that would extend the one-year transition period to a less regulated environment; fairly pay the costs of health professions education; and assure that hospital payment rates for the transition year include all elements of the cost of doing business. While NJHA was successful in lobbying for major improvements to the healthcare delivery system in New Jersey, its advocacy efforts—on behalf of all hospitals statewide—continue to pursue "making the Health Care Reform Act a better bill."

On its 75th anniversary, NJHA is reviewing the past in order to plan the future. Whatever the uncertainty of America's changing healthcare system, one certainty is that New Jersey will provide leadership and innovation.

*A*long with other health-related organizations, NJHA is located at the Center for Health Affairs, which provides an environment for people to learn about and discuss major healthcare issues.
Courtesy, New Jersey Hospital Association

CENTER FOR HEALTH AFFAIRS

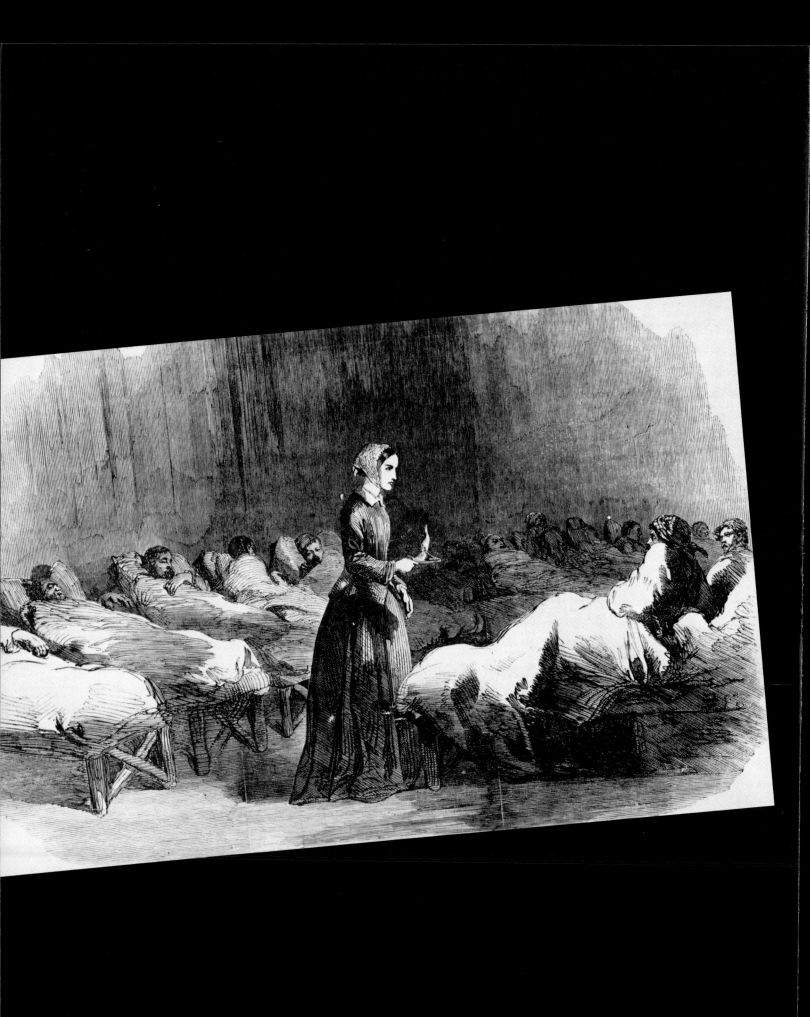

No other institution in America has undergone such a complete transformation as its hospitals. In one century of human history, hospitals evolved from isolated refuges providing custodial care for society's castoffs to complex centers offering the most advanced and specialized medical care to all citizens. The visible aspects—such as physical facilities, equipment, medical procedures, and personnel—bear little resemblance to early hospitals.

Even more fascinating are the invisible, underlying shifts in world views and belief systems that have occurred. Concepts about the nature of humanity, morality, the physical world, and illness, as well as the role of science, religion, social class, and government, have all undergone radical transformations within the 20th century. Because hospitals deal with fundamental human experiences such as birth, death, pain, and caring, they—perhaps more than any other American institution—trace the evolution of thought and belief from the days of the early republic to the modern era.

New Jersey's hospitals have reflected and, by the state's characteristic innovation and inventiveness, advanced this remarkable transformation.

THE EVOLUTION OF HOSPITALS

Custodial Care to Medical Cure

Florence Nightingale (1820–1910) organized a unit of 38 nurses for the Crimean War in 1854, and by war's end she had become a legend. The founder of modern nursing, she created educational systems, changed hospital architecture, and revolutionized methods of hospital care.

Courtesy, The Bettmann Archive

The Origin of Hospitals

Hospitals, defined as institutions to which the sick can be brought for care, existed in ancient civilizations. In Greece and Rome, the temples of the gods served as hospitals where the sick were brought with the hope of cure by divine intervention. Buddha built hospitals for the poor who were crippled or diseased. King Aroha, a monarch in India in the third century B.C., established excellent hospitals known for gentle, humane care. The origin of the modern hospital, however, can be traced to the *hospita*, or hospices, that arose in Europe in the ninth century.

In many ways the early American hospitals of the 18th and especially the 19th centuries bore more resemblance to the hospices of the Middle Ages than to the modern hospitals that emerged in the 20th century. Like the early medieval hospices, the first hospitals in America were an outgrowth of religion, not medicine. They were created out of religious duty as charities for the poor and destitute. They provided comfort, nursing care, and the basic necessities of life, but little in the way of medical treatment, even in terms of the limited understanding and practices of the times. Both medieval hospices—which first appeared along the Crusade routes—and early American hospitals cared for those who were separated from their families.

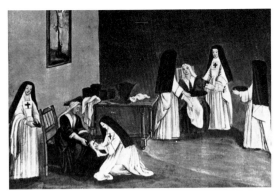

The earliest American hospitals were outgrowths of and reactions to the almshouses. These refuges were founded, out of religious stewardship as well as pragmatic necessity, by the more fortunate and respectable citizens to care for society's dependents: the insane, blind, crippled, orphaned, alcoholic, and economically destitute, as well as those who were injured or ill but had no family to care for them. Although almshouses were established as charities motivated by Christian compassion, conditions were appalling. Filled with society's castoffs—the "depraved and miserable of our race," in the words of a Presbyterian clergyman who ministered to inmates in New York City—almshouses were crowded, filthy, unbearably odorous, noisy, and chaotic. No one entered the almshouse except out of desperation and as a last resort.

Essential to an understanding of the establishment of the first hospitals is the concept, characteristic of the 18th and 19th centuries, of the "deserving" and "undeserving" poor. Almshouses were seen as the rightful place for those whose misfortune was caused by intemperance, moral depravity, or lack of industry. Yet, although the almshouses were the fate "deserved" by the majority of its inhabitants, there were still pious and respectable individuals—especially those struck by illness, injury, or the infirmity of age—whose descent seemed to be not of their own doing. The earliest hospitals in America were intended as alternative care for these worthy poor.

The first general hospital in America was Pennsylvania Hospital, founded in Philadelphia by Quakers in 1752. The second, New York Hospital, was chartered in 1771 but not opened until the 1790s; and the third, Massachusetts General Hospital, opened in Boston in 1821.

Psychiatric hospitals in America have followed a separate course and been subject to different factors. The first mental hospital was founded in Williamsburg, Virginia, in the 1700s, and, in general, mental hospitals were established earlier and evolved apart from general hospitals. The first hospital in New Jersey was the New Jersey Lunatic Asylum at Trenton (now Trenton Psychiatric Hospital), founded in 1848 as a result of the pioneering efforts of Dorothea Dix for humane care for the mentally ill.

The First Hospitals in New Jersey

Until 1863, there were no general hospitals in the entire state of New Jersey. People who were sick or injured recuperated at home, generally under a doctor's supervision and nursed by family members. Those unfortunates who did not have family support or the resources to be cared for at home were often cared for in the local almshouse or pesthouse, which provided shelter to the poor who contracted infectious diseases.

The earliest general hospitals in New Jersey were founded by religious orders in the cities in the north. Urbanization and industrialization were major factors associated with the growth of hospitals. Cities had large numbers of single people—industrial workers or domestic servants—who were cut off from the support of families and small communities. Even where entire, even large, families lived together in poor urban areas, the small, cramped living quarters of tenements made caring for sick or injured family members difficult. Also, the crowded, unsanitary conditions in cities in the 1800s led to outbreaks of such contagious diseases as typhoid, cholera, typhus, and influenza—which could spread to epidemic proportions.

Early 19th-century industrialization was inevitably associated with trauma and injury. An Episcopalian layman asking for hospital funds in *An Appeal for the Sick*, published in Philadelphia in 1851, argued that every steamboat and locomotive meant an increase in injury, and stressed the industrial worker's isolation from family: "The young men employed in our workshops and factories or engaged in the various laborious pursuits which provide the means of living, are generally boarded, at low rates, in small rooms crowded to repletion...." Port cities, especially, were sites of early hospitals because of the necessity of caring for sick or injured seamen far from home.

Many New Jersey hospitals were founded by religious orders. The first acute-care hospital in New Jersey was St. Mary Hospital in Hoboken, founded in 1863 by four Franciscan Sisters of the Poor from Germany. The following year, 1864, the same order sent three additional nuns from Germany to found St. Francis Hospital in Jersey City. In 1867, five Sisters of the Poor began work in Newark's Saint Michael's Hospital, a 13-bed facility that had been fully equipped and furnished by women volunteers working under the direction of the Sisters of Charity. The Sisters of Charity also founded St. Joseph's Hospital for the "sick poor" in Paterson in 1867, St. Francis Hospital in Trenton in 1874, and St. Mary's Hospital in Passaic in 1895. In 1872, St. Peter's Hospital was opened in New Brunswick by Father Miles Duggan, the pastor of St. Peter's Church. It closed in 1874 but reopened in 1907. Saint James Hospital in Newark, now part of Cathedral Healthcare System, opened in 1900 thanks to the generosity of Nicholas Morre, an alderman of the city of Newark and parishioner of Saint James Church, who bequeathed the sum of $25,000 to the parish for the establishment of a hospital and orphan asylum. In 1908 Saint James became the first hospital in New Jersey to perform a blood transfusion. All Saints Hospital, founded in 1892 in Morristown, and St. Mary's Hospital in Orange, founded in 1900, were administered by the Archdiocese of

Newark. Christ Hospital, an Episcopal institution in Jersey City (originally the Hudson County Church Hospital and Home), was founded in 1874 and administered by the Sisters of the Good Shepherd. Alexian Brothers Hospital, purchased by Elizabeth General Medical Center in 1990, was founded in 1892 by brothers from a religious order from Germany. Hackettstown Community Hospital was created through funds raised from the surrounding community and the Seventh Day Adventist Church. The hospital today maintains its religious association under the umbrella of the Adventist Health System.

Ethnic identification and religious affiliation were extremely important to patients in these early hospitals, which served in place of family in times of sickness and vulnerability. In 1865, soon after the first Catholic hospitals opened in New Jersey, six Protestant Episcopal Churches in Newark established Saint Barnabas Medical Center (now located in Livingston, it is presently one of the largest hospitals in the state). In 1871, the Hospital of the Ladies Association (now Wayne General Hospital in Wayne) was established in Paterson as a Protestant response to the creation of St. Joseph's Hospital. At Newark German Hospital, founded in 1868 for the city's large German population, German was spoken and beer was served with meals. Alexian Brothers Hospital in Elizabeth brewed its own beer in the hospital basement for its patients and staff. The Daughters of Israel Hospital and the Hebrew Hospital (now combined to form Newark Beth Israel Hospital), founded in 1901, provided an environment where Hebrew and Yiddish were understood, rabbis visited, and kosher food was served. Nonsectarian Barnert Hospital in Passaic, founded in 1906, allowed Jewish and Italian physicians to practice in the hospital in response to the needs of new immigrants in the surrounding area. Today, Jewish Home and Rehabilitation Center in Jersey City and River Vale provides nursing home and outreach services for frail Jewish elderly. In keeping with Jewish heritage, the center provides care while always making available the ability to incorporate Jewish traditions and moral imperatives into patients' daily life.

After the first religious hospitals were opened, hospitals began to be established by municipalities as a civic duty or by a town's prominent citizens as a source of community pride. Opened in 1868 by the aldermen of Jersey City, Jersey City

Charity Hospital (now Jersey City Medical Center) developed out of what had originally been a pesthouse opened in 1805 for the quarantine of people with contagious diseases. Newark City Hospital, now the University of Medicine and Dentistry of New Jersey-University Hospital, and Trenton City Hospital, now Helene Fuld Medical Center, were founded to offer city residents a general, public hospital in addition to the religious institutions.

Sometimes disease outbreaks or single incidents motivated communities to find the resources for a hospital. For example, the founding of Hackensack Hospital (now Hackensack Medical Center) was motivated by public sentiment and community spirit after a brakeman on the Susquehanna Railroad fell and severely injured his head during the blizzard of 1888. The nearest hospitals were in Jersey City and Paterson, and accounts at the time blamed the delay in reaching Paterson as responsible, at least in part, for the man's death. Long Branch Hospital (now Monmouth Medical Center) began in 1887 by a group of local businessmen when a contagious disease had reached epidemic proportions. Princeton Hospital (now The Medical Center at Princeton) was started by civic-minded citizens during the influenza epidemic of 1918.

Some community hospitals were founded by the philanthropy of one individual. Zurbrugg Memorial Hospital in Riverside, for example, was founded in 1915 with a bequest from Theophilus Zurbrugg, a wealthy watchcase manufacturer. Burdette Tomlin Memorial Hospital in Cape May was built with money (to be matched by area citizens) donated by Burdette Tomlin, a successful retail clothing merchant. Prior to the establishment of Newcomb Hospital in Vineland (now Newcomb Medical Center) in 1924, there had been several failed efforts to maintain hospitals in large private homes in the community. When a campaign was launched in 1919 to raise funds for the construction of a hospital, attorney Leverett Newcomb announced he would contribute $210,000, providing the hospital would bear his name. With his gift and a total of $400,000 raised from the community, the hospital was constructed. Today, Newcomb is a 235-bed hospital serving four counties with services from perinatal care to cardiac rehabilitation.

Often the specialized hospitals of the day were founded because of the appeal of the patients to a founder or to charitable benefactors, as illustrated by each of the four hospitals that merged to become United Hospitals Medical Center in Newark: Crippled Children's Hospital, Babies' Hospital, Presbyterian Hospital, and the Newark Charitable Eye and Ear Infirmary. The Crippled Children's Hospital (now United Hospitals-Orthopedic Center) was founded in 1892 by Samuel Carrach, an

*B*efore the establishment of hospitals and medical centers—as illustrated by an 1870 drawing by C.B. Bush— doctors administered to the ill at home, where they were cared for by family.
Courtesy, The Bettmann Archive

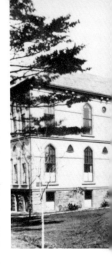

orthopedic brace maker by trade, who was concerned with the plight of homeless crippled children. Babies' Hospital-Coit Memorial was founded in 1909 by Dr. Henry Leber Coit, who formulated a production code for certified milk and improved milk standards in the United States. Presbyterian Hospital was also established as a milk dispensary in 1909, by the Reverend Stubblebine of the Bethany Presbyterian Church. The Newark Charitable Eye and Ear Infirmary appealed to the business community's desire to help working people remain in the work force, when their otherwise untreated medical conditions might lead to blindness or deafness.

The Revolution of Medical Science

Hospitals became cleaner, better ventilated, and more respectable as a result of the experience gained in army hospitals during the Civil War and the teachings of the British nurse Florence Nightingale, based on her experience in the Crimean War. The hospital reform movement in the late 19th century drastically altered the physical aspects and appearance of American hospitals, but the concepts underlying hospitals and medicine remained basically unchanged. Hospitals were paternalistic institutions that reflected a society of class distinctions and social deference. Health and illness were physical manifestations of an all-encompassing moral order. Disease was understood as a general condition—brought on by intemperance, immoderation, or other imbalance—rather than as a specific, localized pathology.

Even though cleanliness and ventilation were essential components of hospital reform, the germ theory was not yet understood or accepted. Most 19th-century physicians as well as laymen believed that a vague, "ferment-inducing" substance in the atmosphere, originating in decayed animal matter and transmitted by the exhalations of the sick, was responsible for hospital infection. Even though anesthesia had been developed in midcentury, few surgical procedures were performed.

There was no medical treatment—including surgery—that could not be performed as well in the home as in a hospital. In fact, medicine and doctors played a very small part in hospital care, which was directed toward providing an environment conducive to the body's natural healing processes. Florence Nightingale, who articulated the common-sense wisdom of the day in her *Notes on Hospitals*, felt that medicine was not a part of the fundamental recuperative process and was useful only in occasionally removing obstacles to healing. Hospital admissions were still based on need rather than on medical diagnosis, and the better-off citizens in society still preferred to be cared for at home in times of illness.

The advance of medical science in general and the germ theory of disease in particular ushered in the modern hospital. Although Joseph Lister had demonstrated the growth of microorganisms in broth in the early 1860s, it was another decade before antiseptic surgery and the germ theory on which it was based became widely accepted. The beginning of the 20th century, however, marked a sharp delineation in the evolution of hospitals. The growth of medical science—with the accompanying reform of medical education and the development of the medical profession—completely transformed the hospital. The germ theory not only expanded the role of surgery, it supported other new concepts in medical thought, such as the specificity of disease. As the germ theory showed a relation between a specific disease or infection and a specific microorganism, disease ceased to be viewed as a general condition that could be manifested as any number of arbitrary outward symptoms.

Scientific medicine gave a new authority to physicians and a new importance to hospitals. By the end of the First World War, the increasing complexity of aseptic surgery (which replaced Lister's antiseptic surgery), the effectiveness of the clinical laboratory, and the development of new equipment such as the X-ray machine made hospitals the focus of medical care. As medical and surgical procedures could now be done in hospitals that could not be done in homes, hospitals became the appropriate and necessary site for the provision of healthcare to the middle and upper classes as well as the poor. Also, although American hospitals—in contrast to those in Europe—have historically had some patients who paid a fee for their care, the early 20th century experienced a revolution caused by the tremendous increase in the number of paying patients. Hospitals entered the market economy.

The Reform of Medical Education

The growth of medical authority was largely the result of the success of science in understanding the world. A common-sense approach to healthcare that depended on order and cleanliness was no longer enough. Nor was a casual, or even a classical, education with little or no clinical training sufficient credentials for a physician. Advances in medical science, many of which came from the large clinical hospitals of Paris and the laboratories of the German-speaking countries, necessitated reform in medical education in America. The American Medical Association, which had grown from 8,000 members in 1900 to 70,000 in 1910, asked the Carnegie Foundation for the Advancement of Teaching to evaluate the nation's medical schools.

Abraham Flexner, a young educator chosen for the task, published his report in 1910. Citing the great discrepancy between medical science and medical education, Flexner's recommendations were straightforward and sweeping. He recommended that all of the first-class medical schools and a few schools from the middle ranks should be raised to the high standards of the Johns Hopkins Medical School, which had joined science and research in clinical hospital practice. The remainder—by far the great majority of America's medical schools—should be closed.

As a result of the landmark *Flexner*

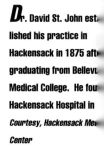

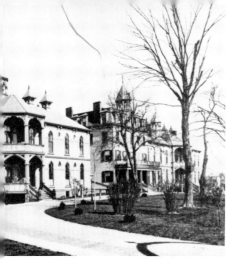

*S*t. Joseph's Hospital and Medical Center, as it looked in the early 1900s, has served the Paterson area for more than a century.
Courtesy, St. Joseph's Hospital and Medical Center

*T*he original St. Peter's Hospital in New Brunswick occupied the Russell mansion from 1907 to 1929.
Courtesy, St. Peter's Medical Center

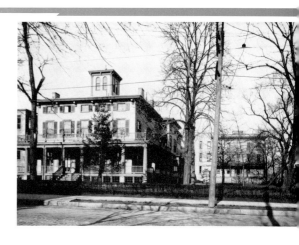

*T*he horse-drawn ambulance was in general use until the 1920s.
Courtesy, University of Medicine and Dentistry of New Jersey–University Hospital

*N*ewark German Hospital, pictured in 1888 in its Newark location, was renamed Clara Maass Medical Center after the humanitarian who gave her life to help develop a yellow fever vaccine.
Courtesy, Clara Maass Medical Center

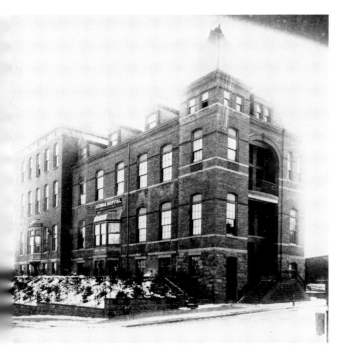

*T*he first Princeton Hospital building was a 1919 farmhouse, located on the grounds of the current Medical Center at Princeton.
Courtesy, The Medical Center at Princeton

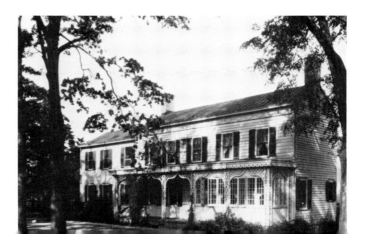

The Emergence of Community Medical Centers

With the advent of the modern hospital as the mecca for the most advanced and specialized medical care in the world—with the astonishing discoveries, procedures, techniques, and cures—came escalating costs, decreased accessibility, and the charge that medical science treated organs and diseases and not the whole person. By the later decades of the 20th century, the hospital needed to become a more flexible institution. Both economics and humanity pointed to a need for regional planning, for expanded outpatient facilities, and for more long-term care facilities. In response, within the last decade America's—and New Jersey's—hospitals have undergone another phase in their evolution. They have become centers in the community, reaching out and offering a variety of ambulatory, preventive, educational, and social programs relating to the well-being of the entire individual.

Report, medical education became scientific, standardized, and hospital-centered. In many ways the hospital became more essential to medical education than the university. The University of Medicine and Dentistry in New Jersey (UMDNJ), in fact, evolved from the Newark City Hospital rather than from a university or medical school. Today UMDNJ is the largest freestanding health sciences university in the United States. Established in 1970 by legislative decree, UMDNJ has an enrollment of more than 3,000 students in a variety of health profession schools located on three campuses across the state. In addition to UMDNJ's own schools, students, interns, and residents are trained in more than 80 affiliated hospitals statewide. An example of New Jersey's innovative leadership, the university was created as an active participant and central force in the state's healthcare system.

As hospitals became "medicalized," physicians played a more prominent and authoritative role in their policies and administration. The traditional authority of lay trustees diminished and status of doctors increased. Once hospitals became more complex, however, new kinds of highly specialized personnel emerged. In addition to nurses, hospitals required professional administrators, technicians, clinicians, pharmacists, dietitians, and social workers. The scientific revolution, which was largely responsible for the emergence of physicians as a sovereign profession, also contributed to the adoption of the professional standards and specialized criteria for a host of other health-related vocations.

Although hospitals are unique, in some ways their evolution followed or paralleled other institutions in society at the beginning of the 20th century. Hospitals, reflecting the new concepts of the times, were changing from "communal" institutions based on the model of the patriarchal family to "associative" institutions based on a new model of professional knowledge and expertise. By the end of the First World War, all of the aspects of the modern hospital were in place: the advances in medical technology; the role in medical education; the professionalism of its personnel; the entrance into the market economy; the increase of paying patients and the establishment of third-party payment; and the beginnings of increased regulation and a larger role for government. Not coincidentally, the New Jersey Hospital Association was established in 1918 as the modern hospital with all its new complexities began to emerge.

New Jersey, with its large urban and elderly populations, has led the country in innovative, hospital-based programs to involve and to meet the changing needs of communities. In 1937, Bergen Pines County Hospital won the American Hospital Association's "National Hospital Day" award for having the greatest community participation in the day's celebration in the entire United States. East Orange General Hospital developed the nation's first Candy Striper program, involving young volunteers from the community in the hospital's patient care. Overlook Hospital in Summit was one of the first hospitals in the country to participate in a national program to establish standards of community service programs. The Memorial Hospital of Salem County was the first hospital in the United States to receive a loan from the Farmer's Home Administration under the Community Facilities Program. Memorial Hospital of Burlington County instituted the first 24-hour emergency room in New Jersey, among the first in the country.

Today, New Jersey hospitals remain in the forefront of addressing community healthcare issues that are social as well as medical. The state's oldest general hospital, St. Mary Hospital in Hoboken, operates the area's largest counseling program for persons with AIDS and their friends and families. In January 1990, the Camden County Department of Health initiated the nation's first program designed to help HIV-positive patients avoid long waits sometimes associated with seeing a doctor. In Camden County, as soon as an HIV-positive status is verified, blood is drawn to determine the condition of the patient's immune system and a Treatment Assessment Program (TAP) begins. A patient can then expect to see a doctor within two to four weeks. TAP, made available through a $40,000 grant from the Camden County Freeholder Board, provides counselors, medical evaluations, case managers, and nutritional services. TAP is located at two sites: UMDNJ School of Osteopathic Medicine in Stratford, serving Kennedy Memorial Hospitals/University Medical Center, and UMDNJ Robert Wood Johnson Medical School in Camden, for Cooper Hospital/University Medical Center.

St. Francis Hospital in Jersey City serves its community with a medical detoxification program. Seabrook House is a multidisciplinary chemical dependency treatment center committed to treating individuals who are suffering from the disease of alcoholism or chemical dependency, their family members, and significant others in their lives. Since 1974, Seabrook House has been working to return troubled individuals to full productivity. Fair Oaks Hospital developed the Outpatient Recovery Centers, which have become a national model for the treatment of substance abuse. Clara Maass Medical Center operates The Safe House, the only known domestic violence shelter in the state affiliated with a hospital. The Woman's Center at Rancocas Hospital offers a full range of services for women throughout their life spans. Hamilton Hospital developed an innovative PromptCare Center designed to treat individuals with non-life-threatening conditions immediately in a setting separate from the hospital's emergency room. Underwood-Memorial Hospital's award-winning paramedic program extends into three counties in rural southern New Jersey and has served as a model program for the state. Betty Bacharach Rehabilitation Hospital opened a Sleep Disorders Center for the diagnosis of sleep apnea and other causes of abnormal sleep patterns. South Jersey Hospital System, a comprehensive healthcare system with hospital divisions in Bridgeton and Millville, offers oncology, hospice, and respite care as well as high-tech cardiac care, renal dialysis, and mental health programs among its many community healthcare services.

Hospital programs now extend far beyond the treatment of the medical condition to treatment of the whole patient, as well as his or her family. The Burn Unit at Saint Barnabas Medical Center features a multidisciplinary approach to burn care that provides emotional, psychological, and family support, in addition to the most advanced medical treatment. Similarly, Cooper Hospital/University Medical Center's cancer program focuses on all aspects of a patient's treatment, including psychological support and rehabilitation. The oncology services of Beth Israel Hospital in Passaic include support and education and are aggregated in one area for staff-patient familiarity and comfort. The Kessler Institute for Rehabilitation offers support groups, peer counseling, a sexuality clinic, driver education, and work-monitoring programs in addition to acute care and physical rehabilitation. Garden State Rehabilitation Hospital in Toms River is another of New Jersey's specialty hospitals. It offers programs for head trauma, spinal cord injury, pain management, and ortho/amputee services. To help meet the needs of families, Ancora Psychiatric Hospital operates the Campus Brief Visit Homes, designed for the use of the patients and their visiting family members. St. Lawrence Rehabilitation Center runs Hotel with Care, a home-away-from-home respite care program that offers services to care for chronically ill or injured individuals when their families must be absent for short time periods.

Today in New Jersey hospitals, there is a growing realization of the human, as well as the medical, dimensions of healthcare. Childbirth, for example, is treated not just as a medical procedure, but as a family experience. Pascack Valley Hospital was the first in the state to offer nurse-midwives admitting privileges and to provide "birth suites" with a birth room, kitchenette, bathroom with shower, and early-labor lounge. Rancocas Hospital was also one of the first New Jersey hospitals to initiate a family-centered approach to maternity care and to offer birthing rooms. The Mercer Medical Center's extensive obstetrical services encourage family-centered births, and nurse-midwives have full hospital privileges. Holy Name Hospital in Teaneck is also known for its comprehensive obstetrical services and family-centered approach. At the other end of the life continuum, Roosevelt Hospital's Barbara E. Cheung Memorial Hospice, the first freestanding hospice in New Jersey, has overnight facilities for family members and a garden on a 1.2-acre wooded site. The Medical Center at Princeton, Riverview Medical Center in Red Bank, the Medical Center of Ocean County, Inc., JFK Johnson Rehabilitation Institute, Southern Ocean County Hospital, and Union Hospital also operate hospice programs.

In 1963, Welkind Rehabilitation Hospital began as the Multiple Sclerosis Home and Treatment Center. During the 1960s and 1970s, the facility continually expanded programs and broadened its mission to serve persons afflicted with various neurological-related disorders. Responding to community needs for a comprehensive rehabilitation hospital, a new 72-bed facility was built in 1984. In 1989, Welkind affiliated with Kessler Rehabilitation Corporation to become part of a comprehensive rehabilitation system serving northern New Jersey.

Some hospitals in the state exclusively serve the needs of children. Founded in 1981, Children's Specialized Hospital—which provides comprehensive services in three locations—has a 100-year-old tradition of caring for children with rehabilitative healthcare needs. The hospital offers acute and long-term care services. The Matheny School in Peapack is a residential and day facility for children and young adults with severe physical disabilities; Matheny specializes in augmentative communications and rehabilitative technology and offers outpatient services as well.

Mental healthcare has moved increasingly from large, state-run institutions to programs in general, community hospitals. In 1933, Elizabeth General Medical Center established the first hospital-based psychiatric unit east of the Mississippi River. Today, it offers a full range of inpatient and outpatient care, including the only inpatient psychiatric unit for children and adolescents in Union and Essex counties. Similarly, the Center for Mental Health of Newton Memorial Hospital is a major mental health facility with a staff of psychiatrists, psychologists, and clinicians. Essex County Hospital Medical Center established the first mental health outpatient clinic in Newark, the first patient remotivation

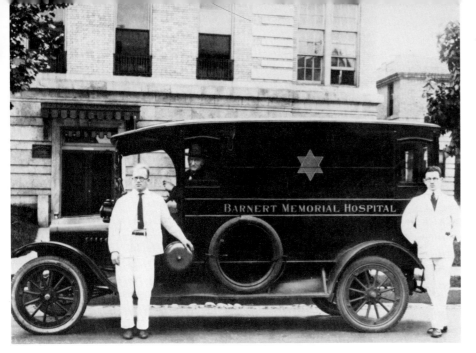

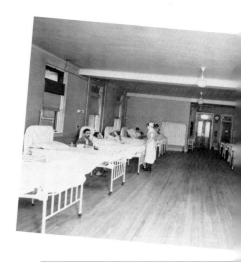

By the 1920s, automobile manufacturers made vehicles specially equipped to transport sick or injured people quickly to the hospital.
Courtesy, Barnert Hospital

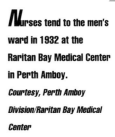

Discovered in 1895 by William Roentgen, X-rays revolutionized doctors' ability to diagnose illness. Morristown Memorial Hospital installed its first X-ray machine in 1903.
Courtesy, Morristown Memorial Hospital

Nurses tend to the men's ward in 1932 at the Raritan Bay Medical Center in Perth Amboy.
Courtesy, Perth Amboy Division/Raritan Bay Medical Center

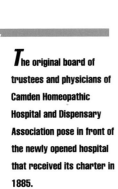

The original board of trustees and physicians of Camden Homeopathic Hospital and Dispensary Association pose in front of the newly opened hospital that received its charter in 1885.
Courtesy, West Jersey Health System

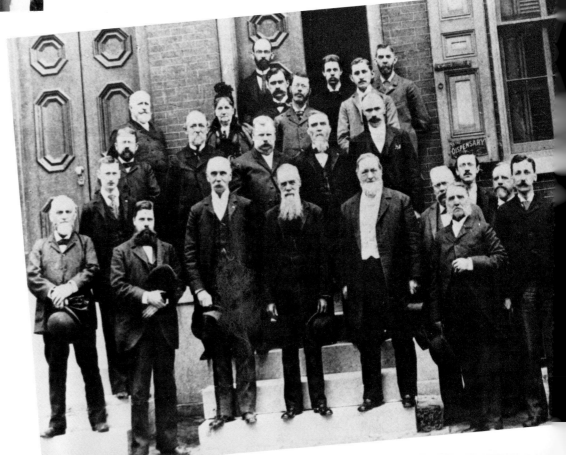

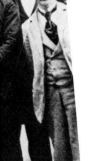

program in New Jersey, and the first joint discharge planning system—now in practice statewide—that coordinates the discharge of psychiatric patients with community agencies and the New Jersey Division of Mental Health and Hospitals. Catholic Community Services offers a psychiatric program that includes detoxification for individuals addicted to opiates, sedatives, or alcohol. Nationally, Essex County Hospital Center was a pioneer in music therapy and established one of the first psychiatric nursing programs in the United States.

Hampton Hospital, a 100-bed private psychiatric hospital located in Rancocas, provides psychiatric treatment, research, education, and diagnostic services for adolescents and adults. Hampton utilizes an interdisciplinary team comprised of a certified psychiatrist, physicians, psychologists, registered nurses, clinical nurse specialists, social workers, certified addiction counselors, and special education teachers, as well as creative, recreational, and occupational therapists in designing and implementing an individualized treatment plan for each patient.

Marlboro Psychiatric Hospital is a public psychiatric hospital that provides care and treatment for the most seriously and chronically ill patients who are unable to be cared for in community settings or private hospitals. The hospital serves adult patients and provides both acute care diagnosis and treatment, as well as long-term rehabilitation of the major psychiatric disorders. It functions as a tertiary referral hospital for the community mental health system. Buttonwood Hospital of Burlington County, located in New Lisbon, also offers psychiatric and long-term care to residents of Burlington County. The 170-bed long-term care division includes two special needs units that address dementia-type programming. The 30-bed psychiatric division cares for patients age 18 and older. Referrals are made for outpatient services. Funding for the hospital is provided by the Board of Chosen Freeholders of Burlington County.

Community Mental Health Center at Piscataway was established in 1972 by UMDNJ. As part of its comprehensive service delivery system, the center operates the only freestanding public specialty short-term psychiatric hospital in the state. Psychiatric inpatient services include a 24-bed acute adult program and a 40-bed child and adolescent unit. In addition, as a pioneer in the establishment of day hospital programs, the center delivers day treatment to preschoolers, children, adolescents, adults, and older adults.

Ramapo Ridge Psychiatric Hospital, a ministry of the Christian Health Care Center founded in 1911, was the first private nonprofit psychiatric facility in New Jersey to provide both inpatient and outpatient treatment for the mentally ill, offering a clear digression from the type of psychiatric care offered in the early 1900s.

Approaches to outpatient and ambulatory services have been especially innovative in many New Jersey hospitals. Chilton Memorial Hospital, for example, was the first hospital in northern New Jersey to offer a mobile mammography service, and Newton Memorial Hospital was one of the first to offer a same-day surgery program. Family Health

Center at Jersey City Medical Center unites all primary-care ambulatory services into a coordinated, comprehensive healthcare system. St. Mary's Hospital in Orange, now St. Mary's Ambulatory Care Center, is the only hospital in the state devoted exclusively to outpatient care, but with the ability to keep patients overnight if necessary. Greenville Hospital in Jersey City has a strong emphasis on same-day surgery, extensively utilizing laparoscopy. The hospital also boasts state-of-the-art ultrasound and mammography equipment, as well as a strong outpatient podiatry program and a family health center that focuses on ambulatory outpatient services for child and adolescent care. East Orange Veterans Affairs Medical Center operates Vietnam Veterans Outreach Centers in Newark and Jersey City and recently opened the James H. Howard Outpatient Clinic in Brick Township. Rahway Hospital, like a growing number of New Jersey hospitals, has publicly stated that it is making a broadened commitment to community ambulatory services and is redesigning its goals, objectives, and courses of action to reflect this redirection.

Newcomb Medical Center, Vineland, recently opened a new Outpatient Cancer Care treatment facility and streamlined its same-day surgery services to allow patients to have a variety of testing and procedures performed in just one visit to the Medical Center. Shoreline Behavioral Health, New Jersey's newest private, not-for-profit psychiatric hospital, opened its doors in August 1992. Services include a full menu of inpatient and outpatient psychiatric and addiction treatment programs.

As for services to the elderly, the Lighthouse of the Community Medical Center in Toms River developed an imaginative, award-winning program that includes a 24-hour toll-free information and referral line, insurance assistance, medical care, and support groups. Warren Hospital offers an assessment and referral program for Warren County's senior citizens. West Hudson Hospital offers long-term care for the elderly, and Palisades General Hospital provides residential care at the Hermitage. The Daughters of Miriam Center for the Aged was the first nursing home in the state to have an ambulatory unit. Zurbrugg Memorial Hospital opened the first hospital-based adult day care center in south Jersey, providing medical supervision, socialization, recreation, meals, and door-to-door transportation. Bayonne Hospital also operates a senior citizen day care center. Bayshore Community Hospital offers the state's most complete array of services for the elderly on a hospital campus: a 180-bed nursing home, 60-bed residential center, and an adult day care center. In its "Vision Statement," the West Jersey Health System articulates this new emphasis of its member hospitals: "Responding to community needs, the System recognizes the growing importance of services for older adults." Grotta Center for Senior Care, located in West Orange, offers community and area residents a full spectrum of nursing and rehabilitation services including short-term rehabilitation and nursing, long-term nursing care, respite care, medical day care, and outpatient services.

Community education and outreach programs

include the Children's Health Fair of Dover General Hospital and Medical Center, which teaches third-graders in local schools about healthy lifestyles. CentraState Medical Center developed a Student Health Awareness Center—the only educational facility of its kind in the state—featuring three-dimensional teaching exhibits and computerized audiovisual displays for area students from kindergarten through high school. Carrier Foundation in Belle Mead, the state's largest private nonprofit psychiatric hospital, using puppets, stories, songs, and art, reaches out to the community with a free program—"Bright Futures for Kids"—offering education and support to children ages 4 to 12 whose families have been affected by alcohol or drug abuse. Elmer Community Hospital offers free health screenings, a weight management program, homebound communications, and a drug and alcohol awareness program for sixth graders. Wallkill Valley Hospital and Health Centers offers an anabolic steroid prevention and education program through Sussex County schools. Columbus Hospital in Newark offers community screenings and health fairs; Somerset Medical Center provides its community with a physician referral information service; and South Amboy Memorial Hospital and Community Mental Health Center provides a speakers bureau.

Several New Jersey hospitals have cooperative arrangements with industry and businesses in the community. The Atlantic City Medical Center established the Atlantic Alliance, a partnership with local business, and Saint James Hospital's Occupational Health Program serves the industrialized "Ironbound" community in Newark. Also, the Outreach Program of Montclair Community Hospital provides a variety of free health screenings—including tests for eye and foot disorders as well as for skin, prostate, and colon cancer—to the community and local businesses. Meadowlands Hospital Medical Center, Secaucus, operates a highly successful Industrial Medicine Center that provides comprehensive health services for business, industry, and government. Among the many services it provides are: emergency treatment of work-related illnesses and injuries and follow-up care; rehabilitation; on-site assessment of health risk factors in the workplace, including asbestos testing; employee drug/alcohol testing; and a wide range of educational programs and seminars. The Meadowlands facility is unique—all its patient rooms are private, in response to studies that show patients in private rooms get more complete rest than those in semi-private rooms or wards.

The Unchanging Mission of Hospitals

For all of the dramatic changes they have experienced during their evolution, hospitals retain an unchanging core of caring. For New Jersey's communities and citizens, hospitals have, in many ways, remained a steady and fixed point. Although the needs of communities have changed, hospitals have been there to meet these changing needs. Perhaps even more important, hospitals have met the unchanging human needs for compassion and respect in times of sickness or injury. The continuity of purpose of New Jersey's hospitals is reflected, and perhaps best expressed, in the words of the mission statements of the hospitals themselves.

St. Mary Hospital in Hoboken—New Jersey's first hospital, founded in 1863—is still "a community of women and men dedicated to the healing ministry....We strive for excellence in providing services to all who need us. We are energized by an atmosphere of joy, mutual respect and compassion to find better ways of serving." Saint Barnabas Medical Center in Livingston, dating from 1864, still strives "in a humanitarian manner to recognize the dignity of all persons and assure those who rely on the Medical Center feel physically, spiritually and emotionally safe and secure." St. Joseph's Hospital and Medical Center, founded in 1867, "holds as a primary value the preservation of the dignity and well-being of man through the promotion, maintenance, and restoration of health." Newark Beth Israel Medical Center, although serving people of any ethnic or religious background, "continues the historic Jewish commitment to service, education and community...deeply rooted in the religious, ethical and social precepts of the Jewish people."

The mission statements of many New Jersey hospitals emphasize that care is to be provided without discrimination and regardless of an individual's ability to pay. Wayne General Hospital, for example, states that the hospital "is committed to meeting healthcare needs...in a compassionate and caring manner...regardless of race, religion, sex, national origin, creed or ability to pay." One hospital's mission statement proclaims simply, "The mission of the Jersey City Medical Center is care-giving. That is its reason for being." Most New Jersey hospitals cite their commitment to the need of the community—or communities—as well as to individuals. Zurbrugg Memorial Hospital in Riverside states, "We believe that our first responsibility is to our patients," but adds, "Our final responsibility is to the community we serve. We pledge to continue in the development of new ideas and innovative programs which will address current and future needs of these communities." The Kessler Institute for Rehabilitation is committed to serving its patients "with compassion and highly personalized care" and also to "meet the healthcare needs of the communities it serves." Dover General Hospital "exists to provide healthcare services which meet the needs of the communities it serves."

Providing care for people in New Jersey's communities is far more complicated today than it was a century ago when all that could be offered was custodial care, kindness, and comfort. Not only have hospitals been the centers of the revolution in healthcare brought about by medical science, they have increasingly become involved in the broader social issues that related to wholeness and well-being. Also, the complex issues facing the healthcare industry today mean that hospitals can no longer "go it alone"; they are interrelated. In a sense, the mission of the New Jersey Hospital Association is the sum of individual missions of its hospitals, and its history is the story of each of theirs. The purpose of NJHA is to ensure that all of New Jersey's hospitals can continue to meet the health and human needs of the people in their communities, as they have done for more than a century.

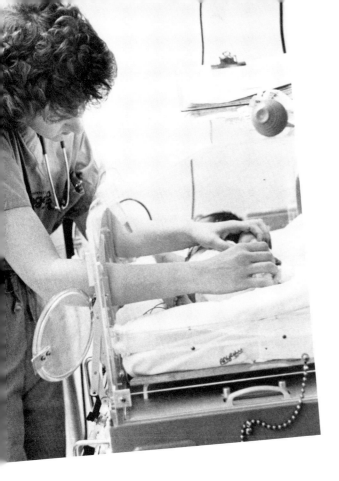

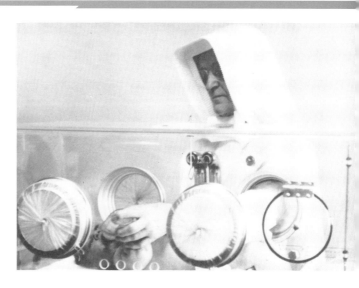

Although technology has changed since its founding in 1905, St. Elizabeth's Hospital recognizes that nurseries have always been shaped by personal attention. A nurse in the 1990s (left) offers the same compassionate care as one nearly 50 years ago (right).

Courtesy, St. Elizabeth Hospital

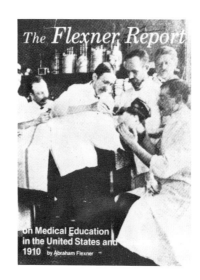

A report by Alexander Flexner initiated sweeping change in medical education by advocating that all medical schools reach the high standards of Johns Hopkins—or close.

Courtesy, New Jersey Hospital Association

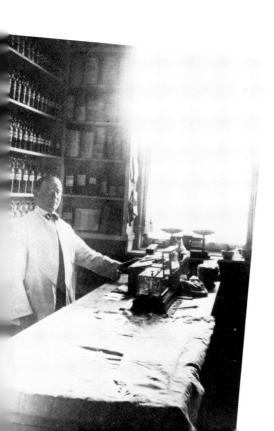

Methods of dispensing pharmaceuticals have changed drastically in this century. An early photo of the pharmacy at Barnert Hospital in Paterson, founded in 1908, contrasts with today's dispensary.

Courtesy, Barnert Hospital

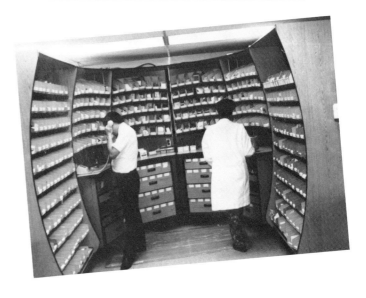

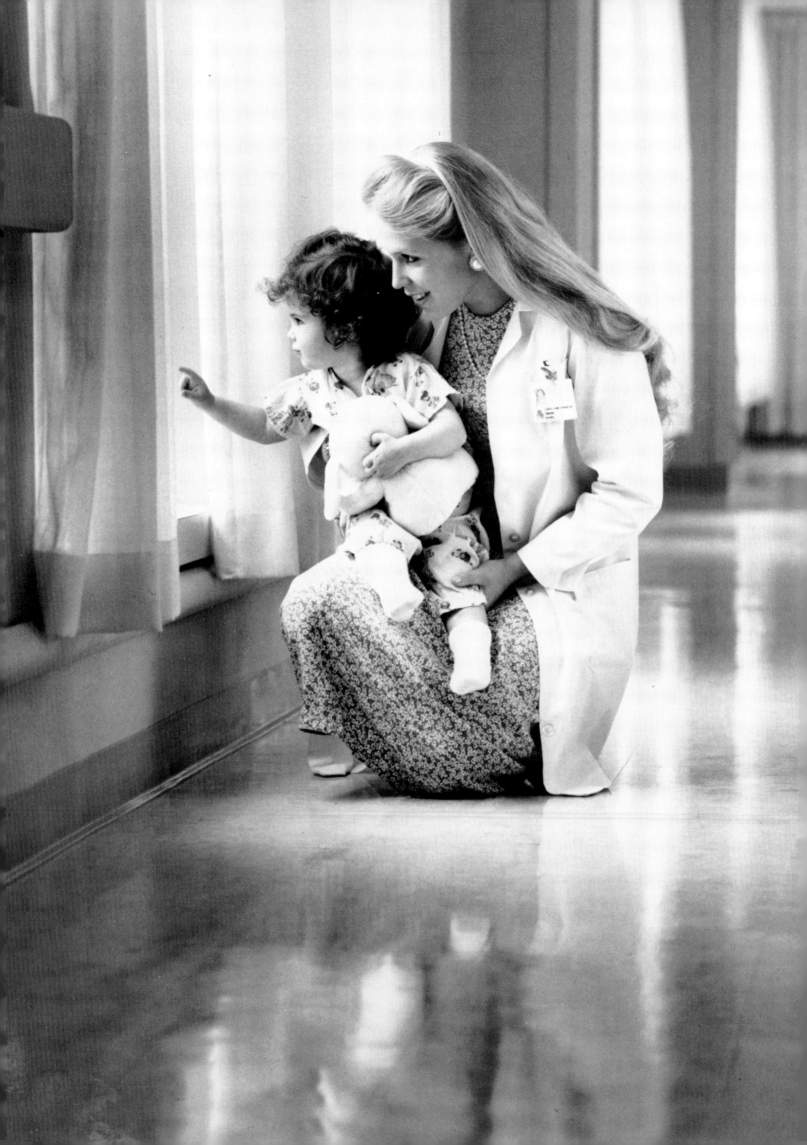

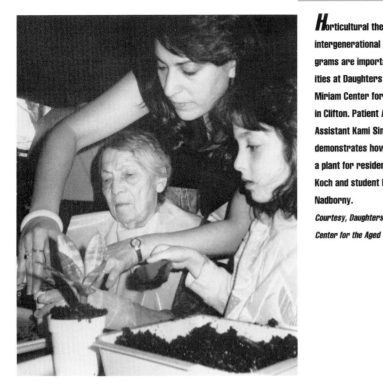

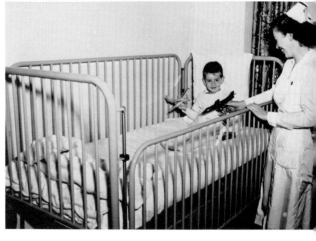

Horticultural therapy and intergenerational programs are important activities at Daughters of Miriam Center for the Aged in Clifton. Patient Activity Assistant Kami Simpson demonstrates how to repot a plant for resident Fanny Koch and student Rivky Nadborny.
Courtesy, Daughters of Miriam Center for the Aged

In 1951, a member of the baby-boom generation enjoyed all the comforts created during the hospital building boom, in newly built Valley Hospital in Ridgewood.
Courtesy, The Valley Hospital

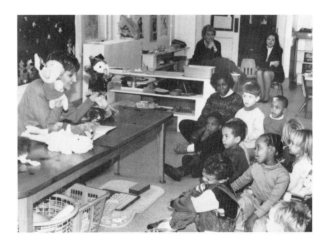

Distracting patients from their illness has been a longtime method of medical care—regardless of their age.
Courtesy, Morristown Memorial Hospital

Students enjoy a program promoting awareness of the dangers of abuse, at Mercer Medical Center's Child Care Center in Trenton—New Jersey's first hospital-based child care center.
Courtesy, Mercer Medical Center

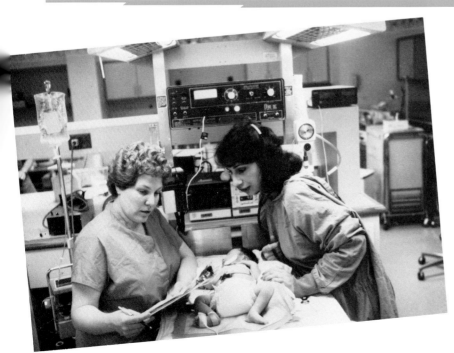

Babies born at West Jersey Hospital–Voorhees in Camden receive care from highly qualified physicians, specialists, and healthcare professionals, and have access to the most modern technologies available.
Courtesy, West Jersey Hospital–Voorhees/West Jersey Health System

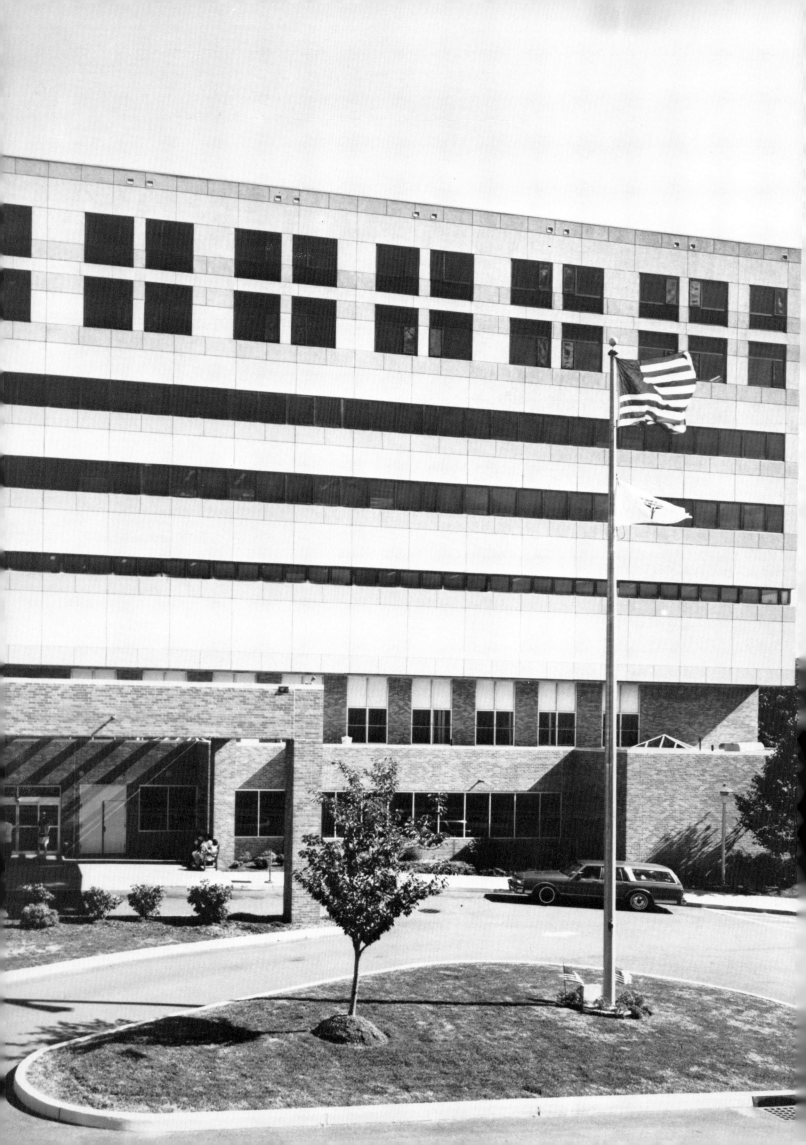

The evolution of ideas that transformed America's—and New Jersey's—hospitals can be seen in the architecture of hospitals through the centuries and decades. In a real sense, the visible physical structures of hospitals reflect the inner, intangible concepts and ideas of medical care.

The *hospita*, or hospices, of the Middle Ages were built, often adjacent to churches, by religious orders that felt called to provide their fellow men food, drink, housing, nursing care, and perhaps even burial. In this Age of Faith, the motivation was religious more than humanitarian. By serving their fellow human beings, the monks and nuns were serving God: "As ye have done it unto the least of these, thy brethren, ye have done it unto me." The typical hospice was more like an inn than a modern hospital, with dining rooms, common areas, and wards.

During the Renaissance—when worldly knowledge was reaffirmed, trade and cities flourished, and life was seen as more than a brief and brutal journey to the hereafter—the hospice evolved into a public service. As a public health measure and civic duty, poor, abandoned, or ill citizens were housed in large structures, still usually run by the church. In fact, the architecture of the *hospita* was often in the shape of a cross, a symbolic reminder of the source of the care. In the still more secular 1700s and 1800s, the Age of Reason, these large public houses—overcrowded with society's castoffs and dependents—were built on a "pavilion" model with independent, connected structures, instead of in the shape of a cross. This design was intended to increase orderliness and ventilation, not so much for the well-being of the inmates but for the comfort of the staff and visitors.

The earliest hospitals in colonial America were not built on as large a scale, but were constructed for the same purpose: to provide custodial care for society's abandoned or homeless sick. America's first hospitals—Pennsylvania Hospital in Philadelphia, New York Hospital, and Massachusetts General Hospital in Boston—were built to separate the physically ill among the "worthy poor" from the almshouse inmates. Like the almshouses, these structures were built as large residences and were conceived of as households managed by a superintendent and his wife. The original rules of the Pennsylvania Hospital, as of many others, required convalescent patients to help in nursing, washing, ironing, and cleaning.

THE ARCHITECTURE OF HOSPITALS

Physical Structures Reflecting Changing Ideas

*S*leek exteriors open to flexible interiors at The Medical Center at Princeton, which dedicates two floors specifically to care for medical/surgical patients.
Photo by Krencicki Photography/The Medical Center at Princeton

The Civil War—a Turning Point for Hospitals

The hospital reforms initiated by Florence Nightingale as a result of her experiences during the Crimean War profoundly affected the organization and structure of hospitals in America as well as in Europe. Her teachings, which advocated cleanliness, spaciousness, and plenty of fresh air, endorsed the "pavilion" style of hospital architecture in which separate wards with windows for cross-ventilation were connected by corridors to common areas. The placement of sewers and drains, and the site of the building itself were designed to maximize the circulation of fresh air—important concerns for mid-19th century planners.

Largely because of the Civil War, America took only a few years to implement the lessons of hospital construction and administration developed by the Europeans during a century of military campaigns. At the beginning of the war, hospitals were extremely inadequate, but improved quickly and steadily. By the time of Lee's surrender in 1865, the Union alone had more than 200 hospitals with almost 137,000 beds. Some of these hospitals built during the war closed after the fighting stopped. For example, in New Jersey, Ward Hospital in Newark opened in 1862 as a hospital for wounded soldiers and closed in 1865.

Not only was there a greater number of hospitals as a result of the Civil War, hospitals had been radically transformed—from large, filthy, chaotic residences for the sick poor to places of active medical treatment. As the Civil War was fought by men from all classes and stations in life, hospitals were no longer for the homeless poor but for the middle class and privileged as well. After the war, the basis for hospital admission continued to be medical, more than economic, need.

As medical science and technology also advanced dramatically during the war, treatments and procedures that could not be performed in homes became available in hospitals. Surgical procedures—along with the use of anesthetics such as ether and nitrous oxide—became well established during the Civil War.

The Industrial Revolution in the late 19th century continued the transformation of hospitals from hospices to diagnostic and treatment centers. Especially in the large, densely populated cities of the North, hospitals were established to handle injuries resulting from industrial accidents as well as the epidemics of infectious diseases.

The First Hospital Structures in New Jersey

The first hospitals in New Jersey appeared in the late 1800s in the industrial cities in the northern part of the state. They were usually established in existing structures, most often large Victorian homes or farmhouses at the edge of the cities. These houses were rented, bought, or donated. Mountainside Hospital in Montclair, for example, opened in 1851 in a rented cottage accommodating 10 beds. Zurbrugg Memorial Hospital in Riverside began in the mansion of its founder. Hackensack Hospital (now Medical Center) started in a 10-room home and barn purchased for $4,000 and later expanded to include the carriage house as well. As in many other hospitals, employees tended a vegetable garden, a herd of cows, and a flock of chickens, and depended on these supplies along with community donations of food for its patients.

Other existing structures were used as well as homes: Long Branch Hospital (now Monmouth Medical Center) began over a delicatessen in rooms rented as a site to care for several children from poor families during an epidemic. A year later the hospital moved to a house with a capacity of six beds, and in 1890, to the Central Hotel, which could accommodate about 100 patients. All Souls' Hospital (now part of Morristown Memorial Hospital) started in the historic Arnold Tavern, which was George Washington's first headquarters when his troops encamped in Morristown during the Revolutionary War. Morristown Memorial Hospital, founded in 1872, opened in a former parsonage that had been built in 1745. Orange Memorial Hospital (now the Hospital Center at Orange) was begun in 1873 in a firehouse and later expanded into a nearby home; in 1882, a new building with 40 beds opened on donated property. Like most New Jersey hospitals, it outgrew its space quickly and repeatedly; a polio epidemic in 1903 even made it necessary for the New Jersey Orthopaedic Hospital (now part of the Hospital Center at Orange) to erect tents in the yard to care for the large number of patients.

A few hospitals opened in buildings specially constructed for them, but these were in the minority in the 19th century. One example is Englewood Hospital in Bergen County, which opened in 1890 in a wooden building accommodating 14 patients, built at a cost of $4,684. St. Francis Medical Center in Trenton began in a four-and-one-half-story building built in 1874; in 1890, a small building was constructed behind the hospital to accommodate patients with contagious diseases.

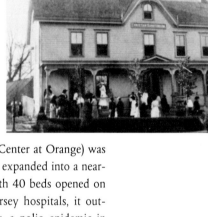

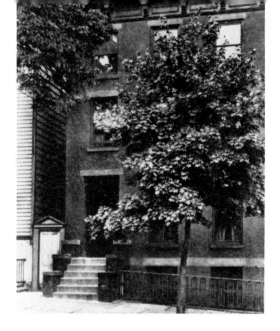

As photographed after it opened in 1867, Saint Michael's Medical Center in Newark celebrated its 125th anniversary in 1992.
Courtesy, Saint Michael's Medical Center/Cathedral Healthcare System, Inc.

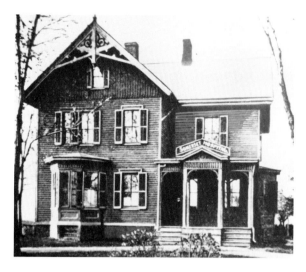

The first building of Somerset Hospital opened its doors in Somerville in 1901 with 12 beds and 10 doctors on staff.
Courtesy, Somerset Medical Center

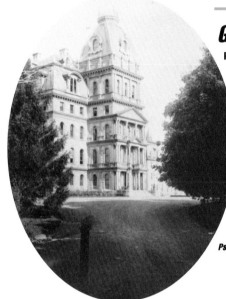

Greystone Park Psychiatric Hospital, as it appeared in the early 1900s, was built in 1876. It had a full basement and the largest single continuous foundation of any building in the country until the Pentagon was built.
Courtesy, Greystone Park Psychiatric Hospital

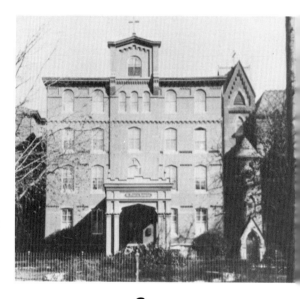

St. Francis Hospital— Trenton's first—was erected in 1874 with donations obtained from house-to-house fund-raising by three nuns.
Courtesy, St. Francis Medical Center

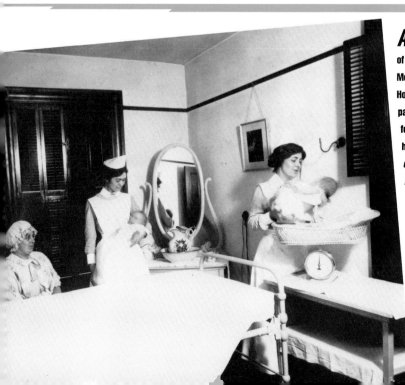

A private maternity room of the early 1900s at Morristown Memorial Hospital catered to patients who would pay for the amenities of a homey atmosphere.
Courtesy, Morristown Memorial Hospital

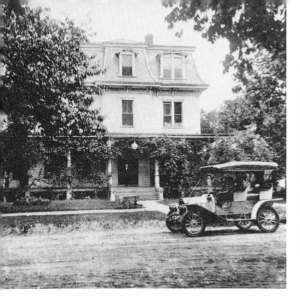

*P*hysicians' Hospital, photographed in 1919, was the Vineland facility used before Leverett Newcomb's financial donation helped build Newcomb Medical Center in the early 1920s.
Courtesy, Newcomb Medical Center

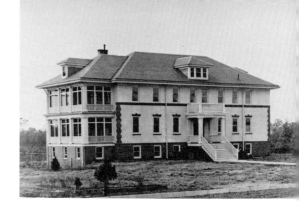

*F*unds for the construction of Millville Hospital were provided by town residents and a matching $10,000 donation from Henry A. Dix. Built in 1915, the hospital featured a 20-bed facility and about 15 staff physicians.
Courtesy, Millville Division/South Jersey Hospital System

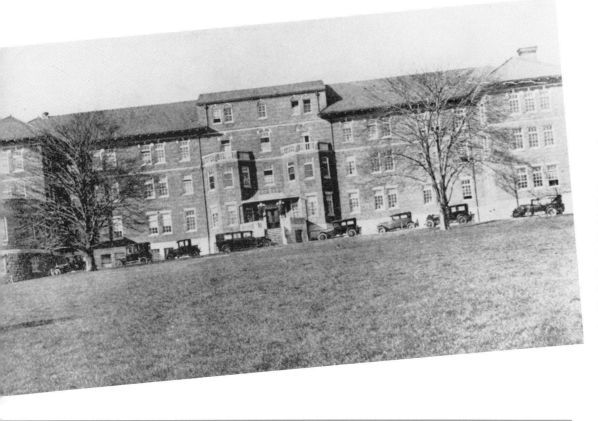

*T*he dedication of surgeons Frank McCormack and George Pitkin, along with Mother General Agatha Brown of the Sisters of St. Joseph of Peace resulted in the opening of the 115-bed Holy Name Hospital in 1925.
Courtesy, Holy Name Hospital

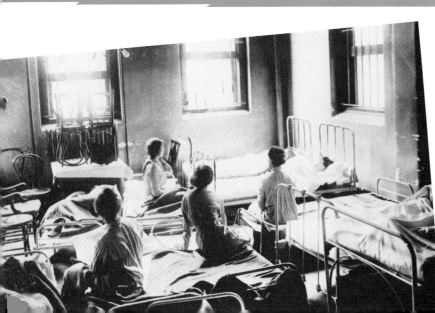

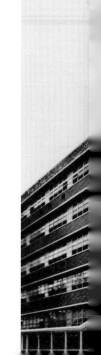

*L*ack of private space in early hospitals led to crowded conditions, as in this women's ward at UMDNJ–University Hospital in 1916.
Courtesy, University of Medicine and Dentistry of New Jersey–University Hospital

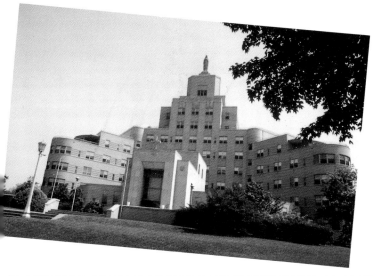

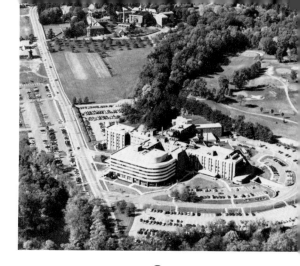

*O*ur Lady of Lourdes Medical Center in Camden was erected in 1950 during the hospital building boom with federal funds sanctioned by the Hill-Burton Act.

Courtesy, Our Lady of Lourdes Medical Center

*S*prawling St Clares*Riverside Medical Center in Denville, founded in 1953, made history as the hospital involved in the landmark Karen Ann Quinlan court case.

*Courtesy, St Clares*Riverside Medical Center*

A long way from its humble beginnings in 1866, Cooper Hospital/University Medical Center serves as the clinical campus for the University of Medicine and Dentistry of New Jersey.

Courtesy, Cooper Hospital/University Medical Center

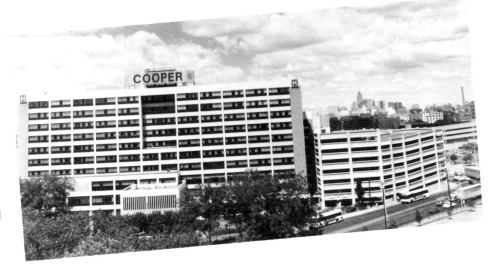

*N*ewark Beth Israel Medical Center is the 10th largest cardiac surgical center in the United States and the site of New Jersey's first heart transplant.

Courtesy, Newark Beth Israel Medical Center

*S*aint James Hospital in Newark continues to provide quality medical care to patients in and around the "Ironbound" section of the city.

Courtesy, Saint James Hospital Division/Cathedral Healthcare System, Inc.

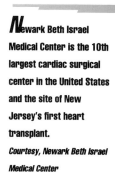

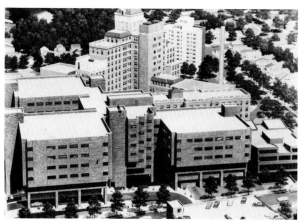

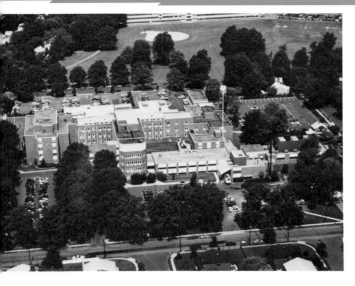

*R*eflective of the ongoing evolution of medical centers in this century, Rahway Hospital, founded in 1916, constantly focuses its emphasis toward community needs. The hospital participates in outreach programs to encourage students to pursue healthcare careers.
Courtesy, Rahway Hospital

*E*xtensive renovation at Jersey Shore Medical Center in Neptune clearly presents the hospital as a high-tech center, where it is known for coronary bypass operations, heart valve replacements, and balloon angioplasty.
Courtesy, Jersey Shore Medical Center

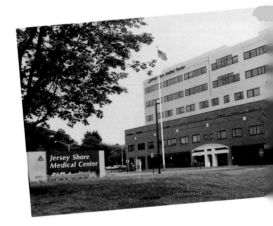

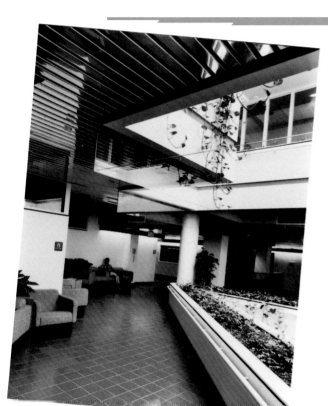

*T*he first-floor lobby of Shore Memorial Hospital in Somers Point exemplifies the trend in hospital architecture toward open space and comfortable waiting areas.
Courtesy, Shore Memorial Hospital

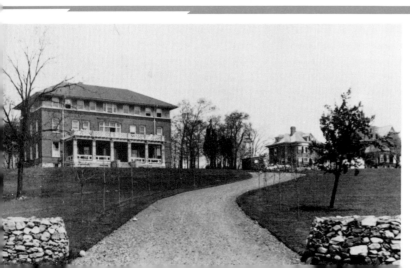

*F*ounded in 1906 with a staff of nine doctors and a horse-drawn ambulance (left), Overlook Hospital has grown to be a 589-bed hospital (right) and is a major teaching affiliate of Columbia University.
Courtesy, Overlook Hospital

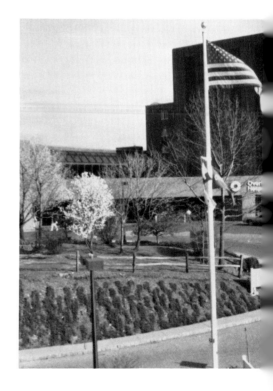

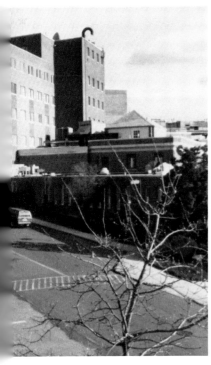

Psychiatric hospitals, which were more concerned with isolation and security, were more likely to be specially constructed. When New Jersey's first mental hospital—built in1848 and now called Trenton Psychiatric Hospital—became severely overcrowded, a second, the New Jersey State Lunatic Asylum (now Greystone Park Psychiatric Hospital), was built in 1876 in Morris County.

In 1910, the 300-acre Belle Mead Farm colony and Sanitorium (now Carrier Foundation) started out as both a farm colony—"a place to produce, purchase, sell and deal in milk, butter, eggs, vegetables, hay, grain and other food, farm, and dairy products;" and colony "for the care and treatment of sick persons, particularly the care of nervous and mental disorders." It was Dr. Russell Carrier who in the 1950s "got rid of the pigs, then the cows, then the chickens—every last one of them." His philosophy: that "mental patients should have the best (care) in the world." In 1956 Dr. Carrier changed the name of the hospital declaring the title *sanitorium* "out-dated and...carries a stigma in the public mind."

Hospital Architecture in the First Half of the 20th Century

By the turn of the century, hospitals were perceived by Americans as acceptable, even desirable, places for medical treatment. Although hospitals in America always had a percentage of paying patients, this percentage increased rapidly in the early 1900s. The fact that occupational distribution of patients became more like that of the general population by the early 20th century is evidence that hospitals served all classes, not just the poor.

This phenomenon was reflected in hospital architecture and structure. Hospitals were designed with smaller, "homier" wards than the airy, utilitarian wards of the large pavilion hospitals endorsed by Florence Nightingale. Newly constructed or expanded hospitals included more private rooms with middle-class comforts and even upper-class amenities. A minority of upper-class patients even had individually decorated hotel-like rooms or suites—with carpets, draperies, easy chairs, paintings, and fine china—that accommodated relatives, nurses, or companions in separate bedrooms. In general, hospitals began by treating the poor for the sake of charity, then added the rich for the sake of revenue, and belatedly designed accommodations for the middle class.

Especially as surgery advanced, more and smaller general hospitals were established in towns and communities to accommodate private patients. These structures were often causes for civic pride and local identity. Often physicians or groups of physicians started hospitals either because they were excluded from existing hospitals or to keep local patients from going to hospitals in large cities.

The advances in surgery and medical technology—which were largely responsible for the new "respectability" of hospitals—affected their structure directly as well. Larger facilities were provided for surgery and new diagnostic equipment, such as the X-ray. Laboratories were built for the newly established clinical sciences of microbiology, chemistry, and hematology. Hospital functions that once all took place in the wards—admitting, diagnosis, cooking, laundry, and even surgery—were now physically separated. As the functions of hospitals became more defined and as standards changed, construction costs increased. The typical hospital in 1870—which had only rudimentary heating and plumbing and was not fireproof—had cost about 15 cents per square foot. In 1905 the same hospital could be built for about 20 cents per square foot, but because of new technological and legal requirements, the actual costs were about 40 cents per square foot.

During World War I, New Jersey's hospitals—especially those in or near the northern port cities—were filled with wounded soldiers. The United States government took over St. Mary Hospital in Hoboken, renaming it Embarkation Hospital Number One (in 1919 it was returned to the Franciscan Sisters of the Poor and again became St. Mary). Although existing hospitals were primarily used during the war, Paterson Army Community Hospital was built in 1919 as a U.S. Army hospital.

After the war, the Veterans Administration built and maintained large hospitals. One of the largest was the Veterans Administration Hospital (now Veterans Affairs Medical Center) in Lyons, New Jersey. Originally constructed as a 400-bed neuropsychiatric hospital in the 1920s, it was expanded throughout the years by additions of both permanent and temporary buildings and could accommodate 2,500 during its peak years.

America, as well as Europe, turned to building a new, modern world. By the 1920s, hospitals, like every other large institutional structure at the time, were being built with electric lights, dynamos, elevators, and mechanized kitchens and laundries. The founding of the American Hospital Association, and of state associations such as the New Jersey Hospital Association, increased professionalism within hospitals and encouraged high and consistent standards; a general consensus emerged as to what constituted a good hospital, in structure as well as in function and organization.

From 1920 to 1940, hospitals grew to accommodate new specialties such as pediatrics and obstetrics. Specialized hospitals emerged as well, such as the Deborah Heart and Lung Center in Browns Mills and the Kessler Rehabilitation Hospital (now one of three facilities that comprise the Kessler Institute for Rehabilitation) in West Orange. Also during this time, the development of penicillin and sulfa drugs virtually eliminated one of the leading killers of hospitalized patients: "hospitalism," or hospital-acquired infections.

New hospitals advertised their sanitation and cleanliness to potential patients. In fact, the efficiency and sterile, no-nonsense "clinicalness" associated with medical science had a tremendous popular appeal to Americans in the early 20th century. Hospital architecture tended to reflect the clear demarcations, efficiency, and functionality appropriate to temples of modern science.

The Growth of Hospitals in the 1950s through the 1980s

World War II, like the Civil War and World War I, brought rapid advancements in medical technology. Not only were new drugs discovered and new surgical procedures developed, but the new understanding of atomic reaction led to the field of nuclear medicine. As the war progressed and more Americans entered battle arenas—and because of the lower mortality rates made possible by antibiotics and surgical techniques—hospitals were filled to overflowing. To meet this need, in 1946, Congress passed the Hospital Survey and Construction Act, popularly known as the Hill-Burton program, to provide federal funds for the construction of community hospitals. Under the law, federal grants provided funds for assessing state and community needs and matching funds up to 50 percent for construction. The landmark federal legislation was responsible for the construction of most of the hospitals in New Jersey and throughout the country.

This period of rapid hospital growth—that included expansions and additions as well as new buildings—occurred primarily in the 1950s through the 1970s. The many hospitals built in all parts of New Jersey during this period include Our Lady of Lourdes Hospital (now Medical Center) in Camden; Burdette Tomlin Memorial Hospital in Cape May; Pascack Valley Hospital in Westwood; William B. Kessler Memorial Hospital in Hammonton; John F. Kennedy Medical Center in Edison; the Freehold Area Hospital (now CentraState Medical Center); and the Bayshore Community Hospital in Holmdel.

The dominant architectural feature of hospitals built during this period was the patient "tower." These high structures, typically built as wings in a T-shape around a central core, were designed to accommodate as many patient beds as possible. Before air-conditioning came into widespread use, the floors comprising the towers allowed cross-ventilation as well as window views. The advent of air-conditioning allowed the use of more internal, windowless rooms, and the towers of patient rooms could be built on a large, flat "pancake" of diagnostic and treatment rooms on the lower levels.

Along with providing funds, the Hill-Burton Act created minimum construction standards to guide architects and planners and to ensure consistency. Many states adopted these standards for all hospitals, not just those built with federal funds. Moreover, although the Hill-Burton guidelines were minimum standards, states often adopted them as maximum construction standards. The long-term legacy of Hill-Burton was immense hospital growth across the country—but construction that was sometimes not of high quality or adaptable to future demands.

In addition to the rapid growth of acute care hospitals, the 1950s also saw increased construction of specialized hospitals, including rehabilitation hospitals, psychiatric hospitals, and Veterans Administration hospitals. These hospitals tended to be larger, more self-sufficient, and more isolated from the surrounding community than general hospitals—in fact, they often constituted their own separate community. Although the Veterans Administration had been founded in 1930, most VA hospitals were built after World War II—often on a grand scale. They provided a comprehensive array of medical, rehabilitative, psychiatric, and social services, and—in the words of Abraham Lincoln—were intended "to care for those who have borne the battle." The first VA hospital to be built in New Jersey was Veterans Affairs Medical Center in Lyons, an acute care hospital with more than 1,000 beds and special programs for post-traumatic stress disorder, head trauma rehabilitation, and Alzheimer's disease, as well as for alcohol and gambling disorders. New Jersey's second VA hospital, the Veterans Affairs Medical Center in East Orange, was completed in 1952 at a cost of $26 million, and has been described—architecturally and functionally—as "a city within a city."

Until the 1960s the federal government's role in hospitals was primarily limited to the construction of their physical facilities. In 1965 the Hill-Burton standards also became a requirement for licensing hospitals qualified to receive Medicaid and Medicare reimbursement.

As these programs grew and the federal government was faced with escalating costs, Congress passed the Health Planning and Resource Development Act in 1974. This new law, which required a Certificate of Need (CN) for new construction, curtailed hospital building and expansion throughout the late 1970s and 1980s.

New Jersey was well prepared to comply with the federal government, since it had passed the Health Care Facilities Planning Act in 1971, which established the CN program and the state department of health as the agency responsible for consistent application of the overall state health plan. According to the 1971 state law: "No healthcare facility shall be constructed or expanded, and no new healthcare service shall be instituted...except upon application for and receipt of a Certificate of Need as provided by this act...."

The Certificate of Need program was introduced to contain hospital costs by preventing unneeded construction or expansion of hospitals. It was reasoned that since hospitals are very expensive to maintain, when beds go unused, the public, in the end, bears the cost of excess capacity. By regionalizing highly sophisticated services such as perinatal care, invasive cardiac diagnostic procedures, cardiac surgery, renal dialysis, and some radiation oncology therapy, these services could be offered more cost effectively. Additionally, as the number of procedures performed by a unit increases, mortality is known to decrease; thus, volume is linked to higher practitioner skill levels and better patient outcomes.

Succinctly stated in the 1988 annual report of the Health Care Facilities Financing Authority, a public corporation involved in helping to secure financing for healthcare construction: "The objectives of the Certificate of Need process are to ensure that: the proposed project will result in high-quality healthcare services; there is a clear and demonstrable need for the project in the area being served; there will be no unnecessary escalation in healthcare costs as a result of this project; and the project is consistent with the goals and objectives of the State Health Plan."

The CN process is complex, until recently involving numerous agencies, organizations, groups and committees—the State Department of Health, the Health Systems Agencies (HSAs), and the Statewide Health Coordinating Council (SHCC), to name a few. Today, the CN process involves input from Local Advisory Boards (replacing HSAs) and the State Health Planning Board (replacing SHCC). If a facility is denied a CN and wants to appeal, the Office of Administrative Law, the Health Care Administration Board, and the Appellate Division of the New Jersey Supreme Court, may become part of the process.

The Challenge of Hospital Architecture Today

The architecture of hospitals has evolved a long way from simple physical structures housing patients. Physical facilities are also no longer viewed as permanent or "cast into stone." Hospitals in the 1990s operate in a highly competitive market economy, with rising costs and ever-changing technology. These factors mean that the design of hospitals today is consumer-driven, cost-effective, and flexible.

Consumer wants and needs are determined by sophisticated marketing research, which is vital to today's hospital planning. Such research indicates, for example, that 70 percent of all admissions are for women and 90 percent of all healthcare decisions are made by women. This finding has important implications for the physical facilities of hospitals, both new construction and renovation. More facilities are designed specifically for women, as well as for geriatric and ambulatory surgery patients.

The general trend is for hospital environments to be homey, convenient, and family-centered. Patient and treatment rooms tend to be painted in soothing neutral or pastel colors (rather than sterile white or "hospital" green) and to have natural or incandescent lighting (rather than fluorescent tubes). Newly designed lobbies feature upholstered furniture, artwork, picture windows, plants, and even fountains or waterfalls. Runnells Specialized Hospital in Union County, one of New Jersey's newer healthcare facilities utilizing modern architecture, offers long-term nursing home care with a distinctly modern atmosphere— the picturesque hilltop facility offers sunlit corridors, spacious courtyards, and gardens.

In addition to changes in the traditional rooms of a hospital, space is allocated to entirely new functions. For example, constructing or modifying areas for educational programs and conferences brings people other than patients and their families into the hospital. Besides meeting community needs, it allows potential consumers to become familiar and comfortable with the hospital. Because more community people use hospital facilities, and because family members are more involved in the care of inpatients, architectural provisions are made for visitors. The courtyard of the Robert Wood Johnson University Hospital in New Brunswick is an excellent example of the use of pedestrian walkways and lounge areas.

In addition to physical attractiveness and comfort, cost is a major consideration in hospital construction today. Good design can enhance the cost effectiveness and operating efficiency of hospitals. For example, new "pod," or "cluster," designs—that keep clinical and support staff in close contact with patients—are much more labor efficient than the long, linear corridors of the traditional T-shaped tower hospitals. The need to house modern technology is another important factor in the physical structures of today's hospitals. Because most of the new equipment is extremely expensive, the trend is to group these resources to provide easy access for the greatest number of people.

Ever-changing consumer needs and rapidly developing technology mean that hospital facilities must be flexible. This is especially challenging for New Jersey hospitals, as they tend to be older than those in most other regions in the country, built with features such as 12-inch-thick plaster walls in a time when little thought was given to future changes.

Today, new or renovated hospital space is carefully planned with flexibility built in, so that when new needs emerge it can be modified without being completely rebuilt. Some of the recent, major hospital construction in New Jersey includes the expansion of the Kennedy Memorial Hospitals–University Medical Center, a three-year, $38 million project that has made it—along with its affiliates in Stratford, Cherry Hill, and Washington Township—one of the largest hospital systems in the state. The extensive renovation projects of The Memorial Hospital of Salem County and Jersey Shore Medical Center in Neptune are examples of modern flexibility and form-follows-function design concepts. The General Hospital Center at Passaic is planning a $27 million building and renovation project. As part of its centennial celebration in 1992, the General Hospital Center Foundation announced a $6 million capital fund-raising campaign.

A century and a quarter after the first hospital opened in New Jersey, the physical structures of hospitals have been transformed as completely as the philosophical concepts that literally shape them. Far from being testaments to permanence, hospital facilities continue to evolve rapidly to meet consumer demands, community needs, and advancing technology. The one constant criterion for hospital architecture is how design and structure can enhance the quality of patient care.

It is not surprising that New Jersey—with its flair for invention and innovation, its location in the highly developed northeastern megalopolis, and its great pharmaceutical companies and burgeoning computer industry—is a pioneer in medical technology. Dating back to its days as a colony, New Jersey's character, spirit, and human resources provided an ideal climate for technological breakthroughs. Its history boasts stories of individuals who have made legendary contributions to the advancement of medical science.

In the 17th century, Dr. William Robinson, a plantation owner in Clark, was one of the first physicians in the colonies to conduct dissection for anatomical study. In the late 19th century, Dr. Henry Leber Coit of Babies Hospital (now Children's Hospital, part of United Hospitals Medical Center in Newark), improved milk standards in the country and formed a production code for certified milk. At the beginning of the 20th century, Clara Maass, a nurse at Newark German Hospital (renamed Clara Maass Medical Center in her honor) sacrificed her life during experiments in Cuba to develop a vaccine for yellow fever. And many of the inventions of New Jersey's own Thomas A. Edison had applications for medical technology.

MEDICAL TECHNOLOGY

New Jersey's Advances and Advantages

New Jersey's Technological "Firsts"

Throughout the 20th century, New Jersey has provided the nation and the world with technological firsts, including:

- The establishment of America's first cardiac clinic in 1926 at Jersey City Medical Center
- The discovery of streptomycin in the 1940s by Nobel Prize winner Dr. Selman Waks of Rutgers University
- The invention of the "New Jersey larynx," which enables victims of throat cancer to speak again
- The development of the "Neville tube," a life-saving prosthetic trachea that creates a new passageway to the lungs
- The pioneering of a method of rebuilding ligaments and tendons with a patented carbon fiber material
- The discovery of the "Armadillo Connection," a link between human and armadillo leprosy, leading to a preventive medicine for people at risk of contracting this ancient scourge, now called Hansen's disease
- The development of effective vaccines for preventing bacterial meningitis, a debilitating and sometimes fatal disease
- The development of a procedure that reduces infection from implants

A computer model of DNA helps scientists establish standards of comparison. Genetic engineering already has become a breakthrough science for diagnosis.
Photo by Howard Sochurek/Medichrome

such as heart valves and arteries by bonding the artificial materials with antibiotics

- The discovery of new drugs that are effective in treating bone marrow infection
- The pioneering use of fluorosol, a blood substitute, for patients who refuse transfusions of real blood because of religious beliefs
- The discovery of a prenatal test for sickle cell anemia, one of the first diagnostic procedures using recombinant DNA technology, or genetic engineering

Many of the state's technological advances are associated with the University of Medicine and Dentistry in New Jersey (UMDNJ), the largest health science university in the nation. Unlike most medical colleges in America, UMDNJ is "freestanding," or unattached to a liberal arts university. The schools that comprise the university are located in Newark, Piscataway, and Camden.

Among the research facilities at the university is the Center for Molecular Medicine and Immunology, established in 1984 to develop proteins that can find and destroy cancer cells. Headed by Dr. David Goldenberg, an internationally renowned pioneer in cancer research, the center is one of the nation's first joint enterprises between a state institution and a private corporation. At the university's Center for Molecular Genetics on the Piscataway campus, some of the world's leading geneticists have been working on advanced research in DNA and diseases of the connective tissue.

UMDNJ's Cancer Research and Treatment Center in Newark, a multidisciplinary facility that opened in 1983, features a million-dollar linear accelerator. The most advanced radiation therapy equipment available, the machine is one of only about half a dozen across the country. UMDNJ–University Hospital also operates a statewide prevention center for high-risk mothers and infants, a regional trauma center, and a regional comprehensive hemophilia care program using the most sophisticated and advanced technology for treatment and care available anywhere in the country.

The Role of New Jersey's Hospitals in Technological Breakthroughs

According to a survey of America's leading surgeons, the greatest technological breakthroughs that have occurred in the 20th century include:
- Computers
- X-rays and CT scanners
- Biocompatible materials
- Respirator/anesthetic equipment
- Endotracheal tubes
- Pacemakers
- Microsurgical instruments
- Amino acid sequencing
- New pharmaceuticals

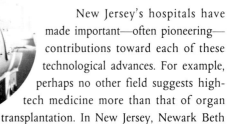

New Jersey's hospitals have made important—often pioneering—contributions toward each of these technological advances. For example, perhaps no other field suggests high-tech medicine more than that of organ transplantation. In New Jersey, Newark Beth Israel Medical Center, the 10th largest cardiac surgical center in the United States, was the site of the state's first heart transplant. New Jersey's first kidney transplants were performed at Saint Barnabas Medical Center in Livingston and Our Lady of Lourdes Medical Center in Camden, which is a regional dialysis and kidney transplantation center. In New Jersey, liver transplants, which are still considered "experimental," are performed only at the University Hospital of the University of Medicine and Dentistry of New Jersey in Newark. St. Joseph's Hospital and Medical Center in Paterson offered the first bone marrow transplants in New Jersey, including autologous grafts, in which patients are the recipients of their own marrow, as well as allogeneic grafts, in which patients receive bone marrow from matched donors.

New Jersey has been a leader in the treatment of cardiac diseases, and two hospitals were pioneers in cardiac surgical procedures. The General Hospital Center at Passaic's cardiac clinic was accepted into the membership of the American Heart Association in 1936. St. Michael's Medical Center, Newark, opened a cardiac clinic in 1937, and a physician at the hospital performed the state's first mitral valve commissurotomy in 1949. In 1958, the state's first open-heart operation—using the heart-lung machine—was performed at The General Hospital Center at Passaic.

Jersey Shore Medical Center in Neptune is a regional center for coronary bypass operations, heart valve replacements, and balloon angioplasty. Newton Memorial Hospital began one of the first cardiac intensive care units in the late 1960s, while William B. Kessler Memorial Hospital was the first hospital in southern New Jersey to have special, advanced cardiac imaging equipment. Hackensack Medical Center has the largest open-heart surgery program of all acute care hospitals in New Jersey. The Heart Institute of St. Francis Medical Center in Trenton offers a complete range of modern preventive, diagnostic, treatment, and rehabilitative cardiac care services. The Cardio-dynamics Department of the Robert Wood Johnson University Hospital in New Brunswick offers a wide range of diagnostic services for heart patients, including echo-cardiology, phonocardiography, and vectorcardiography. A spacious new laboratory for cardiac catheterization was part of a recent building program.

Perhaps New Jersey's best-known cardiac hospital is Deborah Heart and Lung Center, originally founded as a tuberculosis sanatorium in the southern pinelands in 1922. Today

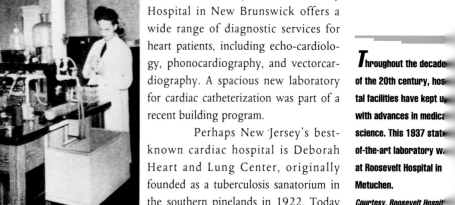

*O*nce known as a miracle of modern science—photographed in the 1930s at Bergen Pines County Hospital in Paramus—the iron lung served as an artificial respirator for victims of polio, or infantile paralysis.

Courtesy, Bergen Pines County Hospital

*T*hroughout the decades of the 20th century, hospital facilities have kept up with advances in medical science. This 1937 state-of-the-art laboratory was at Roosevelt Hospital in Metuchen.

Courtesy, Roosevelt Hospital

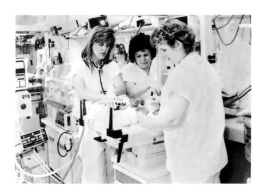

*T*he neonatal intensive care unit of Hackensack Medical Center was started in 1975. It logs more than 3,500 patient days annually.
Courtesy, Hackensack Medical Center

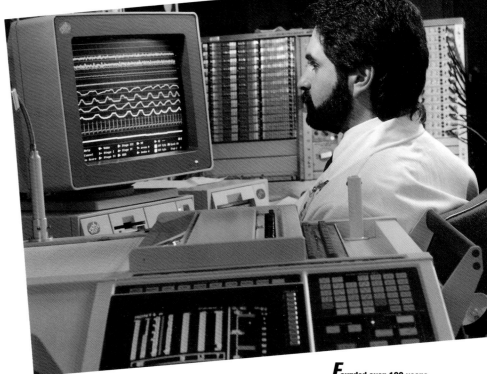

*F*ounded over 100 years ago, Helene Fuld Medical Center boasts electronic equipment to treat sleep disorders.
Photo by Richard Speedy/Helene Fuld Medical Center

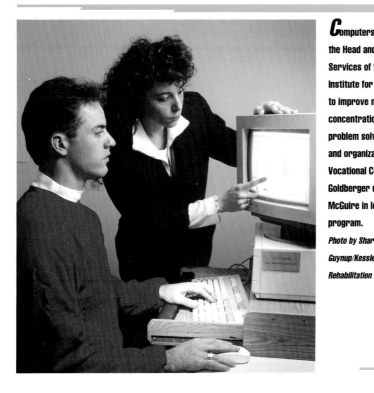

*C*omputers are used by the Head and Injury Services of the Kessler Institute for Rehabilitation to improve memory, concentration, reasoning, problem solving, planning, and organizational skills. Vocational Counselor Cindy Goldberger directs James McGuire in learning a new program.
Photo by Sharon Guynup/Kessler Institute for Rehabilitation

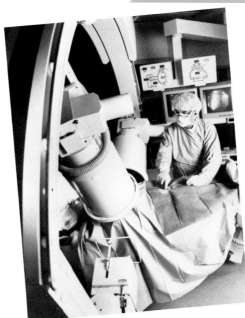

*T*raining in a cardiac catheterization lab has become a standard at Morristown Memorial Hospital's teaching facility.
Courtesy, Morristown Memorial Hospital

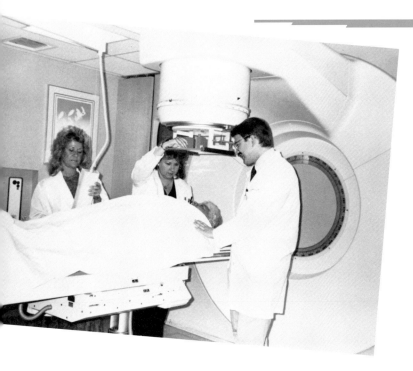

*A*s Director of Radiation Oncology Eli Finkelstein, M.D. (right) positions a patient, senior staff therapists Eve Allegretto (left) and Frances Rey set controls on Elizabeth General Medical Center's linear accelerator. It produces radiation at virtually any level so cancerous cells can be treated with less damage to normal tissue.
Courtesy, Elizabeth General Medical Center

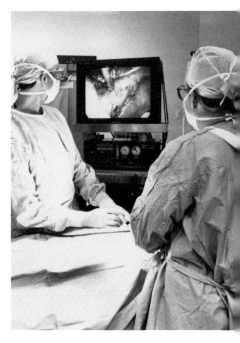

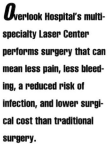

*I*n 1990, Bayshore Community Hospital in Holmdel introduced the KTP laser.
Courtesy, Bayshore Community Hospital

*O*verlook Hospital's multi-specialty Laser Center performs surgery that can mean less pain, less bleeding, a reduced risk of infection, and lower surgical cost than traditional surgery.
Courtesy, Overlook Hospital

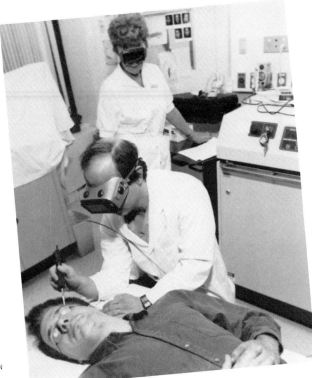

*T*he Skin Laser Center at Pascack Valley Hospital in Westwood offers a variety of treatments, including Copper Vapor, Pigmented Lesion, Q-Switched Ruby, Carbon Dioxide, or Argon lasers.
Courtesy, Pascack Valley Hospital/Well Care Group, Inc.

one of the nation's leading centers for the diagnosis and treatment of heart and lung disease, Deborah is known throughout the world for its humanitarianism and philanthropy. It offers high quality medical and surgical resources at no patient cost.

The Deborah Cardiac Research Institution, which opened in 1981, houses the medical, surgical, and diagnostic departments for the cardiovascular and pulmonary services, as well as Sylvia Martin's Children's World, which treats young patients from all over the world. Among the research fields in which Deborah has been a pioneer is the new field of nuclear cardiology. It was the first medical facility east of the Mississippi to receive the Imatron C-100, a scanner that can make moving and still images of the beating heart.

In the development of medical uses of lasers, Kessler Memorial was the first hospital in southern New Jersey to introduce laser surgery. The first laser spine surgery in New Jersey was performed at the Bayshore Community Hospital in Holmdel in 1972. The Skin Laser Center at Pascack Valley Hospital in Bergen County offers safe, effective treatment of red birthmarks and other benign vascular lesions through the use of copper vapor lasers that beam directly into the affected area. Overlook Hospital in Summit recently opened a comprehensive laser surgery center, staffed by 150 specially trained physicians and nurses.

One of the most useful technological breakthroughs of the 20th century has been the X-ray. Morristown Memorial Hospital installed its first X-ray machine in 1903, only eight years after W. C. Roentgen, a German scientist, discovered the "penetrating rays." Technological descendants of the X-ray that have been developed in recent years include the CT, or computerized topography, scanner. Shore Memorial Hospital and Robert Wood Johnson University Hospital were among the first New Jersey hospitals to install CAT and CT scanners—equipment that is now available to all New Jersey hospitals. Other sophisticated scanning equipment in the state is located at Englewood Hospital's Cytodiagnosis and Breast Cancer Center, an international training site for cytopathology and advanced radiological testing, which features the only mammotest machine in the state.

Perhaps because of its large population of elderly citizens, New Jersey has the largest number of patients with end-stage kidney disease in the country. New Jersey was the second state to establish a dialysis clinic for chronic renal disease patients; currently 2,500 patients receive dialysis at 26 facilities across the state. Holy Name Hospital in Teaneck, which established the first regional dialysis program in northern New Jersey, has been treating patients with end-stage renal disease since 1969. Shore Memorial Hospital was the first known hospital in southern New Jersey to have a chronic renal dialysis center. Saint Barnabas Medical Center, which operates a major regional kidney center, administers dialysis to more than 600 patients each week. Raritan Bay Medical Center's renal dialysis program serves much of central New Jersey, as well as patients from other parts of the state.

In the area of surgical innovations, St. Elizabeth's Hospital in Elizabeth opened the first Intensive Care Unit in 1956. Several New Jersey hospitals have pioneered new high-technology surgical techniques. Wayne General Hospital was one of the first New Jersey hospitals to perform a laparoscopic cholecystectomy—a procedure that removes the gall bladder through small incisions with the aid of a tiny video camera. Burdette Tomlin Memorial Hospital in Cape May was the first hospital in southern New Jersey to perform this new surgery, which is much less invasive than the traditional operation for removing the gall bladder. Recently, thoracic surgeons at St. Peter's Medical Center in New Brunswick devised a similar technique for performing chest surgery. Shore Memorial Hospital in Somers Point has a dedicated noninvasive vascular surgical facility, as well as a state-of-the-art orthopedic operating suite for total joint replacement. Irvington General Hospital, affiliated with Newark Beth Israel Medical Center, is one of only two hospitals on the East Coast that performs gastric banding for morbid obesity. Saint Barnabas Medical Center, a regional surgical referral center, is known for its expertise in microsurgery.

Making High Technology Accessible Across the State

The development and application of new technology in medicine is only half the picture. The delivery of this technology—including issues of accessibility and cost—is the other half. The New Jersey Hospital Association is engaged in long-range planning for the evaluation and delivery of high-technology services across the state, exploring crucial questions such as how high-technology resources should be allocated and how they can be made equally accessible to all New Jerseyans.

In New Jersey, the allocation of high-technology resources occurs after a hospital submits a Certificate of Need and undergoes a thorough review process. In accordance with the New Jersey Health Care Cost Reduction Act of 1991, all existing high-technology resources are identified and monitored by local advisory boards in six state regions. Future resource allocations, however, will match needed services with population, rather than by strict adherence to regional boundaries. Especially in the case of organ transplantation, which is dependent upon the availability of compatible donor organs, a statewide process of allocation may be necessary.

Computerized tomography, an important advance in radiology that allows the imaging of internal structures of the body by computer-assisted X-ray scanning, has proved so essential in diagnosis that it is no longer regionalized. Every major hospital has, or has access to, this equipment. Most other expensive high-technology resources, however, are allocated on a regional basis.

Magnetic resonance imaging (MRI)—which constructs images of an anatomical area based on the reaction of atomic nuclei to magnetic fields—is able to supply diagnostic information that is unavailable from imaging procedures such as CT and ultrasound. In New Jersey, approximately three-quarters of the patients scanned at the state's MRI sites are outpatients.

Another high-technology resource, extracorporeal shock-wave lithotripsy (ESWL), a noninvasive procedure in which electro-hydraulic shock waves pulverize kidney stones, is currently performed at three sites in New Jersey: Mid-Atlantic Kidney Stone Center in Marlton (southern New Jersey), Stone Center of New Jersey/University Lithotripsy Affiliates in Newark (northern New Jersey), and New Jersey Kidney Stone Treatment Center in New Brunswick (central New Jersey). In the late 1980s a similar technique was developed to treat gallstones, called extracorporeal shock-wave biliary lithotripsy (ESWBL). However, the recent introduction of laparoscopic cholecystectomy—the surgical procedure that removes the gall bladder through small incisions—has become the treatment of choice for gallstones.

A major obstacle to the distribution of high-technology equipment and resources in New Jersey is the extensive growth of the nonregulated sector of the healthcare delivery system in recent years. Advances in technology have generally permitted a larger proportion of diagnostic and treatment services to be performed on an outpatient basis in physicians' offices and small facilities unaffiliated with hospitals. This phenomenon has complicated efforts to regionalize high-technology services and ensure reasonable cost.

In addition to state-of-the-art equipment, high-technology surgical procedures, most notably organ transplantation, are carefully allocated and regulated according to regions. Four New Jersey hospitals have organ transplant teams: three have teams for kidney transplants, two for pancreas transplants, and one each for heart and liver. Five hospitals have performed bone marrow transplants.

Organ and tissue transplants are more complex, expensive, and controversial than perhaps any other highly specialized surgical procedure. With the development of new surgical techniques and drugs such as cyclosporine that increase survival by fighting infection and rejection, tremendous advances have been made in the technological aspects of organ transplantation in the last decades.

These procedures, however, involve more issues than the technical challenges. Unlike other medical procedures, transplantation programs depend upon the availability of donor organs and tissues and rely on public education and the coordination of state and national networks and data bases. As often happens in medical science, the social and public issues—such as procurement policies and ethical concerns—have not kept pace with the technological advances.

The Revolution of High Technology of the Future

Most hospital and healthcare observers feel that unparalleled technological advances are just over the horizon. Some feel the future will be so different from anything hospitals have experienced in the past that it will constitute a revolution. Healthcare in the future will be driven by high-technology devices and by consumer demand for that technology. In the coming decades, there will be an explosion of high-technology approaches to the prevention and treatment of disease, especially in the growing area of gerontology. As the life spans of Americans increase, it is likely that the diseases of aging will consume more and more of the nation's healthcare resources and will become the primary focus of medical technology.

These high-technology resources of the future directed increasingly toward an aging population will be of two primary types: biotherapeutics (applying advances in molecular biology) and bioelectronics (using miniaturized computer, or silicon, devices). Some of the possible breakthroughs in molecular biology may include:

- Antibodies that use proteins to help destroy foreign molecules and organisms, including cancer cells
- New vaccines, especially a vaccine for AIDS
- A "tumor necrosis factor" (TNF) that explodes cancer cells
- Gene-spliced proteins to dissolve blood clots
- Gene therapy to identify and correct defective genes
- A substance that will lower blood pressure without side effects
- A DNA probe to identify people with a congenital propensity to form fatty deposits in the arteries
- A diagnostic test that spots early plaque formation in the arteries
- Radioisotope-tagged proteins, called monoclonal antibodies, that can determine the exact site of damage in the heart muscle after a heart attack
- A bioengineering process for producing vitamins
- Eye drops to prevent cataracts
- "Memory pills" to aid victims of Alzheimer's disease
- Brain tissue transplants to treat Parkinson's and other neurological diseases

In the area of bioelectronics, some hospitals will become "body shops" to offer replacement or enhancement of worn body parts. Silicon devices will be increasingly installed inside people rather than outside them; the new field of micromechanics will develop silicon machines so tiny that they can be seen only under a microscope.

An example of this would be the development of a silicon chip that can connect directly to a nerve cell to operate a prosthetic device. Eventually, devices will contain both biological life and silicon surgery working in a synergistic relationship. In cases where technology cannot repair or replace impaired or worn body parts, hospitals will

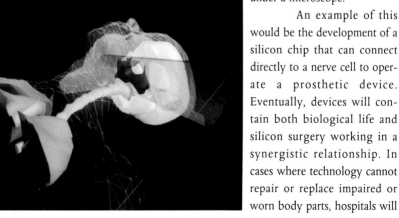

be actively involved in making accommodations to people's living environments. Intelligent robots with a variety of capabilities will be used as "servants" to help people with disabilities.

New technology will create new products, and hospitals will increasingly engage in product development. Physicians, nurses, and other health professionals will spend increasing amounts of time serving on teams that design and develop high-technology medical devices. More and more, hospitals will engage in joint ventures with private agencies and medical groups or will form their own hospital-based multispecialty group practices. Large hospitals will become regional, national, and even international suppliers of their specialized products and procedures. Some futurists in the healthcare field believe that hospitals will begin to look like Silicon Valley corporations—operating on the frontier of high technology, constantly developing new products, and requiring large amounts of venture capital.

What seems certain is that medical technology, escalating in a spiraling progression, will change hospitals to the extent that institutions of the future will have little resemblance to those of today. In a sense, medical technology has already caused a revolution in the history of hospitals, transforming them from residences providing custodial care for the homeless poor to centers providing medical treatment to all classes of society. It may well be that technology will revolutionize hospitals once again. If so, New Jersey's hospitals are well positioned to be leaders in this second technological revolution.

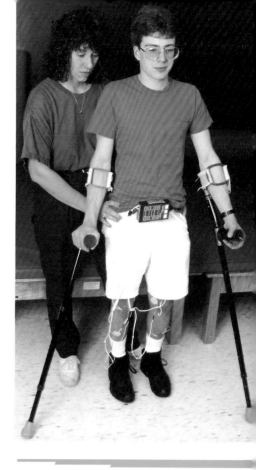

Sue Schweer, associate director of outpatient physical therapy at Kessler Institute for Rehabilitation, guides Chris Britton as he uses a computer-controlled Parastep system to walk. Functional Electrical Stimulation (FES) enables certain patients to exercise paralyzed legs.
Photo by Sharon Guynup/Kessler Institute for Rehabilitation

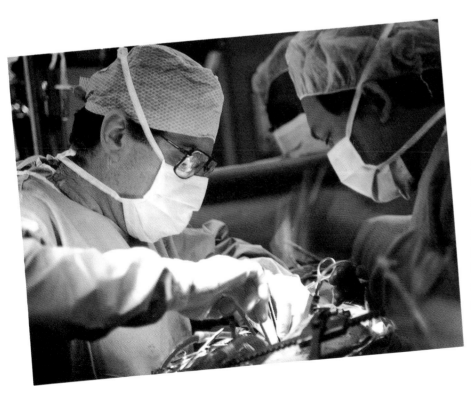

St. Joseph's Hospital and Medical Center in Paterson now performs surgical procedures undreamed of when the facility was founded in 1867. Many patients can return home the same day.
Courtesy, St. Joseph's Hospital and Medical Center

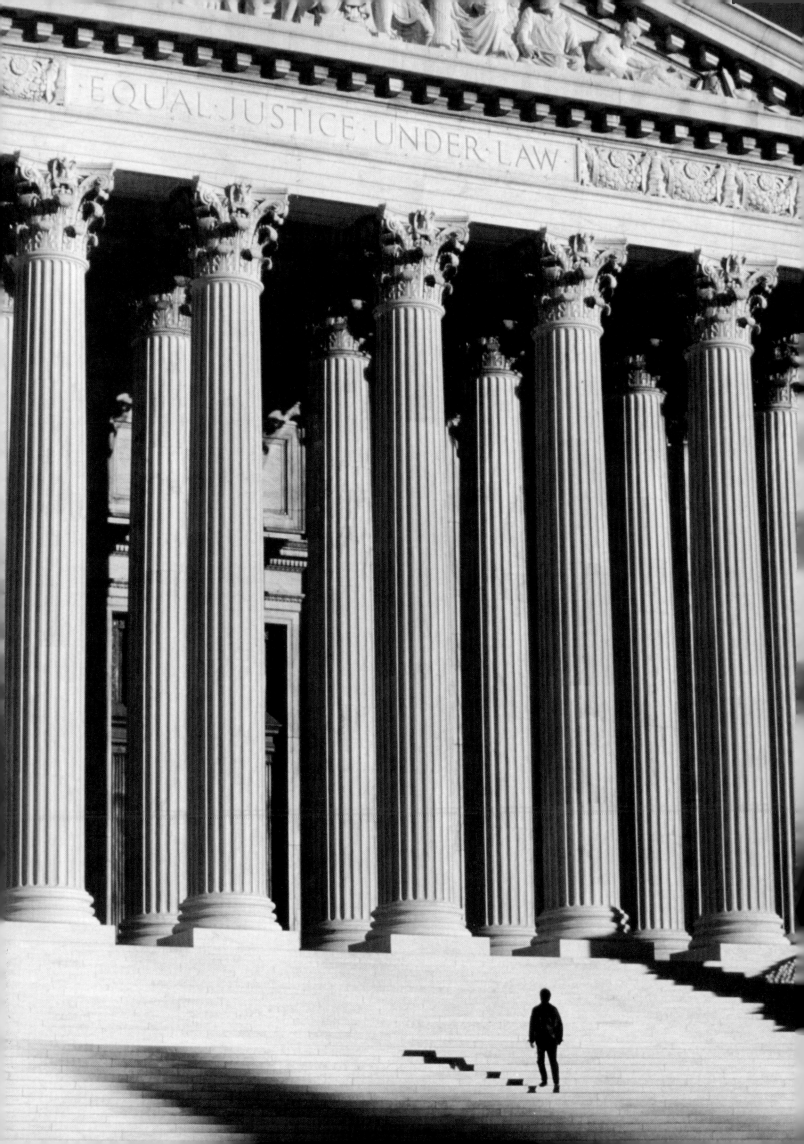

M edical ethics, no less than medical technology, has undergone a revolution in the lifetime of most Americans. Amazingly, the history of medical ethics can be divided into two periods, the traditional era of physician paternalism, lasting thousands of years, and the new era of patient autonomy, dating from only the mid-1960s.

The Era of Paternalism

Traditionally, throughout almost all of human history, medical ethics was the province of the physician and related solely to the physician-patient relationship. A model of paternalism, this relationship was characterized by integrity and knowledge on the part of the physician and trust and gratitude on the part of the patient. The ethical standards governing the physician's role in this relationship were given formal expression in the Hippocratic Oath, written in the fourth century B.C. and still used in some medical schools today:

"The regimen I adopt shall be for the benefit of my patients according to my ability and judgment, and not for their hurt or any wrong. I will give no deadly drug to any, though it be asked of me, nor will I counsel such.... Whatsoever house I enter, there will I go for the benefit of the sick, refraining from all wrongdoing or corruption.... Whatsoever things I see, in my attendance on the sick or even apart therefrom, which ought not to be noised abroad, I will keep silent thereon, counting such things to be as sacred secrets."

Hippocrates also admonished physicians to perform their duties "calmly and adroitly, concealing most things from the patient while you are attending to him...comfort with solicitude and attention, revealing nothing of the patient's future or present condition."

For thousands of years, medical ethics was conceptualized and written by physicians. Just as medicine became a field apart from the sciences and humanities—and increasingly from daily human affairs—medical ethics grew separately from the broader philosophical discipline of ethics.

From the classical age onward, the most distinguishing feature of medical ethics was the extent to which it was the domain of physicians, not philosophers. Except for Roman Catholic moral theology—which applies church doctrine to medical questions for those within the Catholic fold—there is a curious silence about medical ethics in traditional ethical

PATERNALISM TO AUTONOMY

The Revolution in Medical Ethics

M any issues of patients' rights are decided by the United States Supreme Court as medical ethics evolve from the exclusive domain of the physician to include the legal system and Congress.

Photo by Mark E. Gibson

literature. Unlike the ethics of philosophy, which reasons from general principles or "first causes," medical ethics has a decidedly practical rather than theoretical bent. In fact, many treatises—dealing with correct behavior in the community, the patient's home, or at the bedside—sound more like medical etiquette than medical ethics.

As medicine has generally been practiced and taught in an empirical, case-by-case, hands-on manner, it is not surprising that the ethics articulated and transmitted by physicians have the same characteristics. It is telling that, until very recently, medical ethics was not taught in the classroom but on the ward, by medical students emulating their teachers—practicing physicians.

The writings and teachings of medical ethics spell out the obligations of physicians that required them to act not only responsibly, but virtuously. To cite an example in the United States, in 1801 Benjamin Rush, a Philadelphia physician and signer of the Declaration of Independence, in a series of lectures on the "vices and virtues of physicians," admonished that the care of patients came before "ease, convivial company, or public amusements or pursuits."

The physician was to be self-denying to the point of heroism. If an epidemic struck, for example, the physician's duty was to stay and treat the sick, at the risk of his own life. The ethical standards of the medical profession clearly required the physician's selfless duty to the patient, even though the physician did not always live up to them (during the plagues of the Middle Ages there are accounts of physicians shouting instructions outside of fortified walls to monks treating the stricken within).

The traditional view of the sanctity of the physician-patient relationship was stated as recently as 1969—actually after the forces that caused the revolution in medical ethics had been set in place—by the philosopher Hans Jonas: "The physician is obligated to the patient and to no one else. …We may speak of a sacred trust; strictly by its terms, the doctor is, as it were, alone with the patient and God."

Thus, physicians shared a powerful tradition of professional ethics that went back to centuries before Christ and continued through the first half of the 20th century. In the 1920s and 1930s, when major changes were occurring in medical delivery and technology, the American Medical Association insisted that medical ethics (and therefore medical policy) should be left entirely to the physician. The AMA appealed to the timeless ethic based on the physician-patient relationship to oppose a variety of new policies such as health insurance and group practice.

During the 1940s, the medical discoveries facilitated by the war—such as the efficient production of penicillin and vaccines for influenza and typhoid—enhanced the stature and reputation of the medical profession (the atrocities associated with medical research in Nazi Germany were viewed as irrelevant to medical ethics in the United States). In the 1950s, in the popular culture of this calm decade, Marcus Welby, M.D. symbolized the kindly, beneficent family doctor who always "knew best."

Although medical achievements throughout the traditional era of medical ethics were comparatively modest, the paternalistic model dealt well with the psychological aspects of disease. Even if physicians could not effect a cure, they could provide personal care and comfort. During this period, medicine emphasized the power of information. Only physicians knew the prognosis, which they imparted selectively at their discretion. Also, as technology was limited, the physician's personal relationship with the patient—and often the patient's family as well—provided the best clues for diagnosis.

In this era, which many people long for nostalgically, medical ethics was concerned with the relationship between the physician and the patient; few outsiders penetrated this private, even sacred realm. In spite of the inequality implicit in this relationship and the limitations of medical science, the paternalistic model addressed and satisfied many basic human needs in times of illness and suffering throughout the centuries.

The Roots of the Revolution in Medical Ethics

A revolution in medical ethics, completely transforming the relationship between the physician and patient, occurred within one decade. This period of critical change began with the scandals in human experimentation that came to the public's awareness in 1966 and culminated with the case of Karen Ann Quinlan, the New Jersey Supreme Court's landmark decision affirming patient autonomy, in 1976.

In the space of these 10 years, the patient rather than the physician became the authority on his or her own "best interest." Physicians—who for thousands of years had ruled uncontested in their private domain—now had to share decision-making in the public arena, with patients, bioethicists, sociologists, clergy, administrators, lawyers, judges, legislators, and citizens in the community.

The upheavals that led to this new era began, not in medical practice, but in medical research. In 1966, the American public was outraged by an article written by a Harvard Medical School professor, Henry Beecher, and published in the New England Journal of Medicine, citing abuses in human experimentation. The article documented 22 projects, including experiments in which mentally retarded residents of a state institution were infected with hepatitis and elderly, incompetent patients were injected with cancer cells. In almost all of the cases, the subjects would not benefit and might be harmed. Moreover, patient consent had not been obtained—or even perceived as a consideration.

Yet as unconscionable as the experiments seemed, they were not bizarre, isolated examples but were representative, even typical, of the large-scale medical research establishment that began—with public endorsement—during World War II. Between 1941 and 1945, medical research grew from a cottage industry, in which individual physicians performed experiments (usually on themselves, their families, or their neighbors and with a beneficial, or at least beneficent intent) to a well-funded national program involving teams of professionals.

Medical experiments that once had the aim of ben-

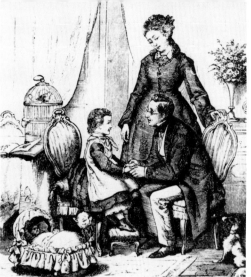

efiting the subject were now intended to benefit others: soldiers on the battlefront. The common understanding that experimentation required the consent of the subject was overridden by the urgency of war. Moreover, as all civilians were expected to make sacrifices for the war effort, participation in medical research by institutionalized populations (orphans, mentally impaired persons, and prisoners) seemed to be an appropriate way of their contributing to the common good. Experiments were conducted to treat dysentery, malaria, influenza, venereal diseases, and to deal with physical hardships such as sleep deprivation and exposure to cold temperatures.

After the war, however, medical research continued and expanded with little oversight or interference, following the utilitarian rules of wartime. The 20-year period between the close of World War II and the publication of Dr. Beecher's article has even been called the Gilded Age of Research. (The Nuremberg Code for human experimentation requiring the voluntary consent of human subjects—a result of the Nuremberg trials held in Europe during this period— was not upheld in American research. If anything, the Nazi atrocities reinforced America's feelings that government should not be involved in medical research.)

After the publication of Dr. Beecher's exposé, the United States quickly became a leader among industrialized nations in the regulation of human experimentation. The National Institutes of Health promulgated comprehensive guidelines covering all federally funded research involving human experimentation and introduced the critical element of public-policy review. The new regulations and oversight recognized that the primary principle of medical ethics— physicians should act only for the well-being of their patients—must hold for the researcher as well.

Soon afterward, physicians at the bedside as well as researchers in the laboratory would come under scrutiny, review, and regulation. Almost immediately after the scandal in human experimentation came the breakthroughs in organ transplantation, first with kidneys in 1966 and then, in 1968, hearts. The reluctance to trust researchers to protect the well-being of their subjects sometimes turned to an unwillingness to trust physicians to protect the well-being of their patients.

The possibilities of conflicts of interest were too apparent. The treating physicians might be more concerned with the long-range benefits to society from perfecting a transplant procedure; the benefits to the patient in the next room needing a new heart; or perhaps even the benefits to their own professional career and reputation. Heart transplantation also involved the issue of scarcity of resources, as had kidney dialysis, developed in the early 1960s.

These technological advances illustrated the inadequacy of the traditional way of dealing with scarcity (usually

on the battlefield)—triage. This concept called for those who would most benefit from medical treatment to be treated, not those who would die with or without treatment, nor those who would live, with or without treatment. Yet in cases of kidney dialysis or organ transplantation, the choices must be made among patients who would all die without medical intervention. This called for criteria other than strictly medical.

Recognizing this, one of the first ethics committees in the nation was formed in the state of Washington, composed of laypeople as well as physicians, to decide who would receive dialysis and who would not (who would live and who would die). After physicians eliminated patients on the basis of medical criteria, the committee evaluated the potential organ recipients on nonmedical criteria, preferring the married over the single, the parent over the childless, the employed over the unemployed, the churchgoer over the nonchurchgoer. While the guidelines of social respectability of this early committee have been criticized (one critic pointed out that Henry David Thoreau would have been summarily rejected for dialysis because of his lack of contribution to society according to conventional criteria), the idea of a group, rather than an individual, making difficult decisions has continued.

The astonishing advances in medical technology—such as kidney dialysis, organ transplantation, and the artificial respirator—are often cited as the reason for the revolution in medical ethics that wrested decision-making power and discretion from physicians. Certainly there has been the widespread perception that science and technology have far outpaced the medical profession's ability to deal with the resulting human and social implications—and ethical dilemmas. Still, the growth of medical technology alone probably could not have precipitated the revolution in medical ethics. Conceivably, if the trust had not been eroded, physicians could well have been perceived as the experts who knew best how to use the new technology.

At least as important as the burgeoning technology in bringing about the revolution in medical ethics—and closely associated with the loss of trust—was the social activism of the 1960s. The uproar

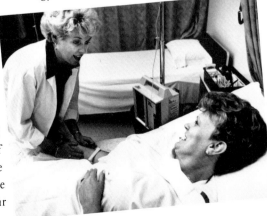

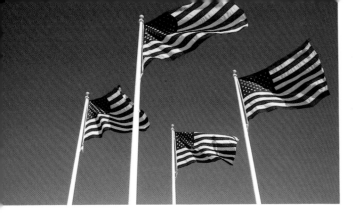

who conducted the hearings, observed that "human experimentation is part of the routine practice of medicine." As a result of the Kennedy hearings, Congress created the National Commission for the Protection of Human Subjects, consisting of 11 members chosen from the fields of ethics, theology, the physical sciences, the social sciences, and the humanities, as well as medicine. In 1978, the commission became the President's Commission for the Study of Ethical Problems in Medicine and at last had the scope that some members of Congress had urged a decade before.

Instances of abuses in human experimentation continued to surface in the 1960s and early 1970s; the most widely publicized case was that of black men in Tuskegee, Alabama, who were not treated for syphilis in order to study the long-term effects of the disease. Increasingly, however, another kind of case involving medical ethics began to attract public attention: that of handicapped newborns who were not given medical treatment.

Johns Hopkins, one of the country's preeminent teaching hospitals, was among the first to establish an ethical review board, in response to the controversy over a baby born with Down's Syndrome who was not treated for an intestinal blockage. Also partially in response to the case of the "Johns Hopkins baby"—which had attracted the interest of the Kennedy family—Georgetown University founded the Kennedy Institute, to join biology with ethics in what is now called bioethics. A similar think tank, the Hastings Institute, was established in New York. Like the President's Commission, these institutes and hospital review boards included members from other disciplines besides medicine. Never again would medical ethics be the exclusive domain of physicians.

over human experimentation became linked to the rights movements that were gaining strength, largely because the great majority of research subjects were drawn from racial or ethnic minorities, the poor, or the mentally disabled. The concepts of personhood and autonomy championed by the Civil Rights Movement, the Peace Movement, and the Women's Movement were antithetical to the paternalism and authoritarianism of the traditional, physician-dominated medical ethics. Increasingly, physicians not only had to deal with a bewildering array of forms, committees, and medical outsiders, but with more assertive, self-determined patients as well.

Commissioning Ethics

In 1968 Congress joined the ranks of the medical outsiders who had become interested in questions of medical ethics. Three months after the world's first heart transplant had been performed by Dr. Christiaan Barnard in Cape Town, South Africa, Walter Mondale, then a senator from Minnesota, introduced a bill to establish a Commission for Health Sciences and Society to assess the implications of biomedical advances. Stating that "the scientific breakthroughs of the last few months…and others yet to come raised grave and fundamental ethical and legal questions for our society," Senator Mondale felt that it was essential to create a national commission with representation by laymen as well as physicians. Dr. Henry Beecher, the Harvard Medical School professor who had blown the whistle on abuses in human experimentation, concurred: "Laypeople must bring their own ethical rules to medicine because science is not the highest value under which other values have to be subordinated." Testifying at the hearings held to establish the commission, Dr. Beecher recalled the words of the atomic scientist J. Robert Oppenheimer: "What is technically sweet, though irresistible, is not necessarily good."

Yet the proposal to establish a national commission was vigorously opposed by most physicians (Dr. Christiaan Barnard was among those who testified at the hearings) and did not pass. The hearings impressed upon the American public, however, that the feats made possible by advances in medical technology had transferred medicine from the category of a helping profession to the category of engineering. Also, at its leading edge, medical practice was much closer to medical experimentation than it had been in the past—and should probably be subjected to the same kinds of oversight and scrutiny.

Indeed, when the proposal to establish a commission was reintroduced in 1973, Senator Edward Kennedy,

New Jersey's Judicial Leadership—the Karen Ann Quinlan Case

The culmination of the decades-long process that transformed the medical ethics of paternalism to the bioethics of patient rights culminated in the New Jersey Supreme Court decision in the case of Karen Ann Quinlan. Its impact on national policy far outweighed the scandals in human experimentation and the death of a disabled newborn at Johns Hopkins. The decision consolidated the trends of the preceding decades and set the framework for subsequent court decisions and legislation across the country. As a result of the *Quinlan* case, New Jersey became recognized as a national leader in

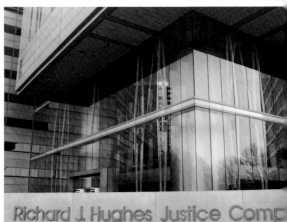

Richard J. Hughes Justice Comp

addressing the ethical and legal dilemmas posed by advances in medical science and technology and in affirming the rights of the patient.

The facts of the *Quinlan* case are well known. In 1975, the young woman, who had lapsed into a coma after ingesting alcohol and drugs, was brought to St Clares *Riverside Medical Center in Denville. When St Clares denied the request of her parents to remove Karen, who was in a "persistent vegetative state," from a respirator, the parents appealed to first the New Jersey Superior Court and then to the New Jersey Supreme Court, which heard the case. The Court made the Quinlans the guardians of their daughter and allowed her to be taken off of the respirator. (She did not die, however, but lived for several years in a long-term care facility.)

In making the case for the Quinlans, Paul Armstrong, who later served as the chairman of the New Jersey Bioethics Commission, centered on Karen's (and her surrogate's) constitutional right to determine her own medical care. Invoking the centuries-old tradition of medical ethics, the state attorney general argued that "no court... should require a physician to act in derogation of the sacred and time-honored (Hippocratic) oath." Yet, within the space of one decade, that view no longer held. The *Quinlan* case firmly established the principle that the patient (or the patient's surrogate), not the physician, is entitled to decide whether or not to pursue treatment.

The case of *Nancy Beth Cruzan v. The Missouri Department of Health* was the most publicized of the more than 50 right-to-die cases brought since *Quinlan*. Cruzan was a 32-year-old woman, reduced to a persistent vegetative state by automobile injury. In *Cruzan* the U.S. Supreme Court endorsed the concept which had been first articulated in New Jersey, that of a patient's constitutionally protected right to refuse treatment.

The New Jersey Supreme Court has subsequently built on the *Quinlan* case in four opinions, continuing New Jersey's reputation as a national leader. The court's decision in the case of Claire Conroy in 1985 is widely acknowledged as a landmark decision, as it extended medical intervention to include artificially provided nutrition and hydration. A trilogy of cases—those concerning Kathleen Farrell, Hilda Peter, and Nancy Jobes—heard by the court in 1987 further established a patient's right to refuse or terminate treatment. Although the circumstances of the patients differed—Farrell was a competent adult being treated at home; Peter, an elderly incompetent patient being treated in a nursing home; and Jobes, a young, mentally incompetent nursing home patient—the court recognized that all patients have a general constitutional right to privacy that encompasses the more specific right to refuse medical care. This right applies whether the patient is competent or incompetent, young or old.

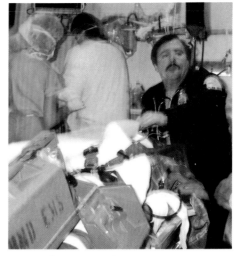

Legislating Morality

After the *Quinlan* decision, legislatures entered the area of medical ethics, typically to the end of expanding patient choices and narrowing physician discretion. The number of cases being heard by courts across the country indicated a need for legislative guidelines, especially laws to define death and to provide for patients who want to express their wishes while competent (by means of advance directives such as living wills).

The definition of death as "brain death," first defined by a Harvard Medical School committee in 1968 and adopted by the President's Commission for the Study of Ethical Problems in Medicine and Biomedical and Behavioral Research, became widely accepted by the medical and legal communities and by the American public. The President's Commission recommended that the determination of death be addressed at the state level, but urged that all states adopt a uniform statute in determining death.

New Jersey's brain death legislation, while it defines death—like other state statutes—as the cessation of function of the entire brain, is unique in that it provides an exemption from this definition if this would violate the patient's personal religious beliefs. In respect for New Jersey's diverse, pluralistic population, the law allows for a determination of death according to the traditional standard of cessation of heartbeat and breathing for individuals (such as Orthodox Jews) whose religion defines death in those terms.

In regard to legislation concerning advanced directives, a few months after the *Quinlan* decision, California enacted a "living will" statute. Other states as well as the federal government, with the Patient Self-Determination Act, followed. New Jersey's 1991 Advance Directives for Health Care Act is grounded in the basic commitment—set forth in New Jersey Supreme Court decisions—that patients should

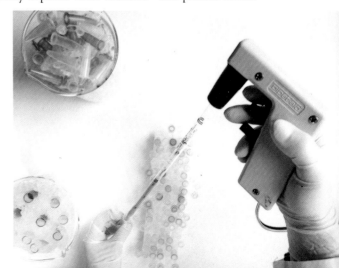

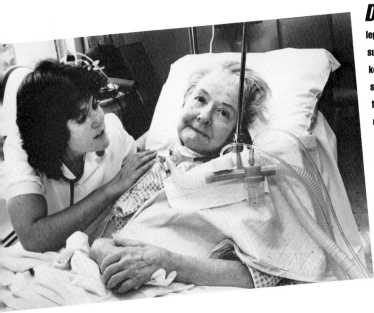

*D*ue to recent legislation, patients—such as this woman being kept alive on a life-support system—have the right to control decisions about the extent of their medical treatment.
Photo by David M. Grossman

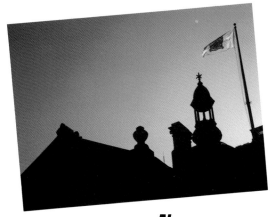

*N*JHA increasingly works with legislators of the New Jersey Statehouse to maintain a balance among medical technology, ethics, and issues of hospital responsibilities.
Photo by Rebecca Barger

*H*ealthcare professionals at Mountainside Hospital benefit from the wide variety of educational resources and activities available in dealing with today's biomedical issues.
Courtesy, Mountainside Hospital

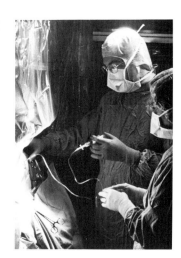

*E*ven when unable to communicate their wishes, patients and their families are empowered with fundamental rights that allow them—not their physicians—to make choices about life-sustaining medical technology.
Photo by David M. Grossman

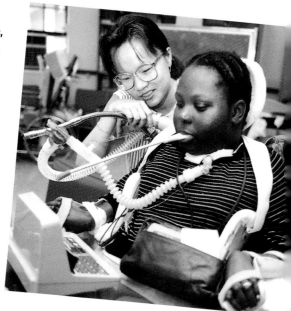

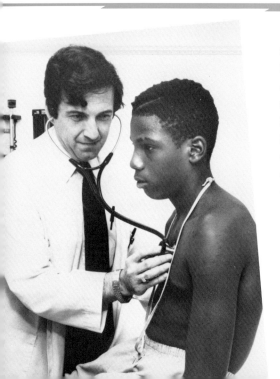

*W*alk-in healthcare centers, such as Health Park One at Saint Mary's Ambulatory Care Hospital, are focusing on keeping patients well by offering preventive services.
Courtesy, Saint Mary's Hospital/Cathedral Healthcare System, Inc.

*S*t. Joseph's Hospital and Medical Center in Paterson performed the first bone marrow transplants in New Jersey. The hospital has a committee for ethical discussions concerning Catholic tradition and patients' rights.
Courtesy, St. Joseph's Hospital and Medical Center

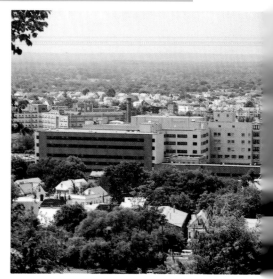

not lose their fundamental right to control decisions about their own medical treatment because serious illness or injury makes them unable to communicate their wishes.

On the Front Lines—Ethics Committees

Bioethics may seem at times to be an ephemeral enterprise, conducted in academic halls and judicial or legislative chambers. Yet it is a human, everyday endeavor, as well. The front lines, where the theoretical dictums of philosophy and formal pronouncements of legislation are applied to real-life people and situations, are the ethics committees.

The New Jersey Hospital Association's Ethics Committee, founded in 1985, works closely with the Medical Society of New Jersey, the Citizens Committee on Biomedical Ethics, the Bioethics Committee of the Medical Society of New Jersey, and the ethics committees of each of New Jersey's hospitals. In 1991, these groups collaboratively amended legislation that became known as the New Jersey Advance Directives for Health Care Act. This law provided citizens the right to outline in advance choices regarding decisions at the end of life. The NJHA Ethics Committee helps develop policies and procedures, sponsors conferences and seminars on bioethical issues, and provides educational resources for hospitals and healthcare professionals. To keep New Jersey's hospitals informed of developments in the rapidly changing area of ethics, the committee publishes a newsletter, *Bioethics Update*, and a routinely updated bioethics reference manual.

In 1991, the NJHA Bioethics Committee, with the University of Medicine and Dentistry of New Jersey, conducted a survey of hospital ethics committees in New Jersey. The findings indicated that all New Jersey acute care hospitals had or were currently forming an ethics (sometimes called a prognosis) committee. Forty-three percent had ethics committees for more than six years, 45 percent from two to four years, and only 12 percent for less than a year. "Ethical needs" was given most often as the reason for the committee; "clinical needs" ranked second; and the "*Quinlan* decision" ranked third. Ethics committees devote most of their time (45 percent) to clinical case review and consultation, 33 percent to institutional policy, and 15 percent to educational and informational programs.

According to the survey, the average New Jersey hospital ethics committee is composed of 14 or more members, and all committees are multidisciplinary. Members include physicians, nurses, hospital administrators, trustees, attorneys, risk managers, dietitians, respiratory therapists, psychologists, gerontologists, patient representatives, community representatives, and bioethicists.

Several New Jersey hospitals have been pioneers in applying bioethics and in developing bioethics committees and policies. Overlook Hospital in Summit has made groundbreaking contributions to bioethics in New Jersey, including sponsoring a conference of federal and state advance directive legislation. The Mountainside Hospital in Montclair offers a variety of resources and activities to edu-

cate healthcare professionals in biomedical issues. St. Joseph's Hospital and Medical Center in Paterson is a excellent example of a Catholic hospital that has formed a proactive multidisciplinary ethics committee that serves as a forum for ethical discussions affirming Catholic tradition and the new rights of the individual. The Valley Hospital in Ridgewood, through its expanded pastoral care program and Biomedical Ethics Committee, has been in the forefront in addressing medical ethics and treating the "whole" of its patients. The hospital has long recognized pastoral care as an integral part of the treatment process and has worked for many years with local clergy through an Advisory Council to the Chaplaincy, designed to respond to increasing needs of patients. In particular, the principles and practices of organ and tissue donation at The Valley Hospital have contributed to its emergence as a leader in this area. The hospital's organ donation program had been operating 15 years before New Jersey's "assured option" law of 1987, which mandates that all hospitals must offer patients' family members the choice of donating organs whenever the donation is medically possible.

The Future of Bioethics and Medical Decision-Making

In the not-too-distant future, escalating medical technology will pose new ethical dilemmas in issues such as physician-assisted dying, the allocation of scarce resources, and surrogate parenting. The "Baby M" decision again brought the New Jersey Supreme Court into the national spotlight. The court found the surrogate contract to be in conflict with New Jersey law and public policy and therefore voided the lower court's termination of the surrogate mother's parental rights. It granted custody of the baby to Mr. Stern, Baby M's natural father, but also mandated "unsupervised, uninterrupted, and liberal visitation" between Baby M and her birth mother. Debate over surrogate parenting may become especially critical in the next few decades. Both traditional physician-centered medical ethics and the recent patient-centered bioethics focus on the benefit to the individual patient rather than on society at large.

As medical care becomes more and more costly, ethical decisions may have to be made concerning the reimbursement for, availability of—and even rationing of—medical resources. Some futurists feel that the time may come when society cannot give each individual what he or she may want or need for optimal health and longevity, and at the same time, have everything else needed to make a good society. America, which spends a greater percentage of its gross national product on healthcare than any other industrialized nation, may not be able to pay for an expanding healthcare system based on the increasingly sophisticated and expensive marvels of medical technology.

Yet, rather than physician discretion, patient rights will be the guiding principle, even if they must be balanced more in the future with the collective rights of society. Bioethical decisions will continue to be made in the public arena—a concern not only of physicians, but of all citizens.

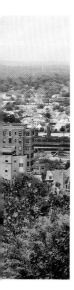

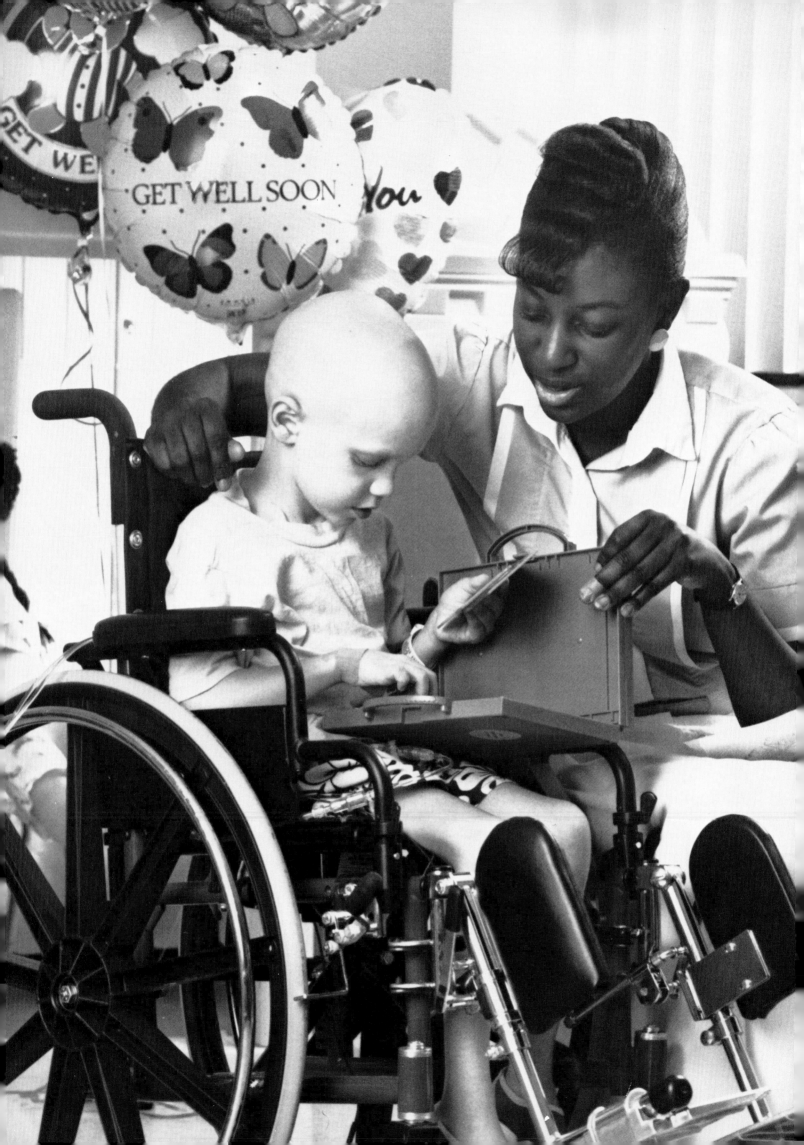

Commitment to quality is the very foundation on which hospitals have been built. In fact, most hospitals and healthcare facilities would probably describe themselves in terms of the quality of care they provide their patients.

Even though quality is at the core of the mission and purpose of hospitals, and even though patients and hospital staff feel they know when it is or isn't provided, the concept of quality has resisted precise definition. Only a few decades ago it was customary to avoid debates on quality by asserting that the concept was too elusive to define. Today it is no longer defensible or feasible to judge quality on an intuitive basis. Quality, in order to be improved, must be defined and must be measured.

Defining quality may be like trying to hit a moving target, but it is essential. The definitions developed by healthcare organizations and agencies—while they may seem rather circular—are a start. The American Medical Association defines quality care as care "which consistently contributes to improvement or maintenance of the quality and/or duration of life." The definition of quality by the Joint Commission on the Accreditation of Healthcare Organizations is "the degree of adherence to generally recognized contemporary standards of good practice and achievement of anticipated outcomes for a particular service, procedure, diagnosis, or clinical problem." For individual hospitals, quality can mean accreditation, committees, peer review, risk management, and patient surveys. A quality program can include all of these activities, and many more.

But quality is more than the sum of its parts. Today, quality is viewed as an all-encompassing, all-pervasive way of thinking that involves all staff, all procedures, and all planning. The concept of total quality that is being newly adopted by hospitals is an exciting concept that is not only fostering first-rate patient care, but helping to contain costs by reducing waste, duplication of effort, inefficiency, and low employee morale.

QUALITY AS CONTINUUM

The Commitment to Quality Care

Lisa Moragne, R.N., talks with patient Scott Merulla in the child therapy playroom at Cooper Hospital/University Medical Center.
Photo by Eugene Mopsik/Cooper Hospital/University Medical Center

The Evolution of Quality Improvement in Healthcare

The idea of quality—as good care and appropriate treatment producing good outcomes of health and recovery for the patient—is as old as the art and science of medicine. The modern concept of "total quality management," or "continuous quality improvement," is a recent construct, but one that evolved naturally as quality indicators began to be actually measured rather than merely intuited.

The prominent hospital reformer, Florence Nightingale, also was a

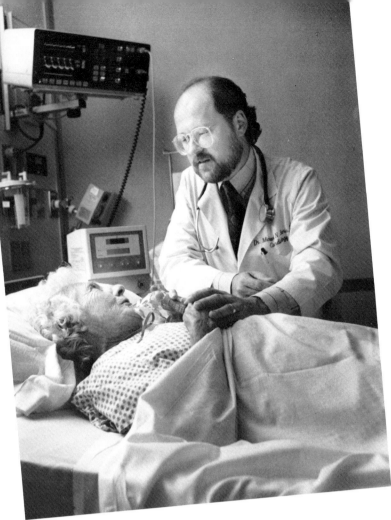

Cardiologist Michael N. Boriss visits a patient at Burdette Tomlin Memorial Hospital.
Photo by Craig Terry/Burdette Tomlin Memorial Hospital

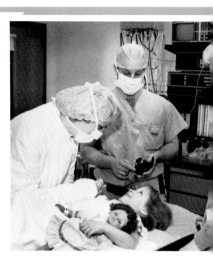

By allowing parents to accompany their child into surgery, Overlook Hospital can ease a young patient's mind and turn an unfamiliar experience into a comfortable, hand-holding one.
Courtesy, Overlook Hospital

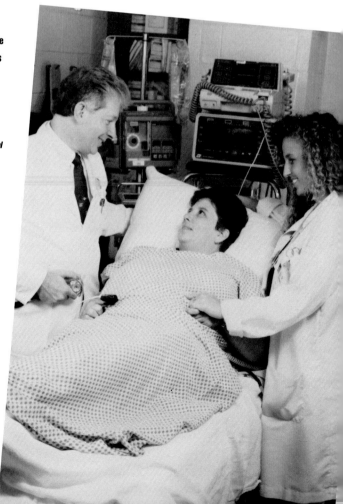

A patient in the emergency room of Shore Memorial Hospital agrees to a doctor's recommendations for treatment.
Photo by Enrosia Photography/Shore Memorial Hospital

pioneer in collecting and analyzing statistical data. During the Crimean War in the mid-19th century, Nightingale recorded the mortality rates of British soldiers, dividing the total number of hospital deaths by the diagnosis category. She used these numbers to illustrate that improvements in sanitation reduced fatalities and increased recovery rates.

In 1842, a less well-known British subject, Edwin Chadwick, conducted a survey to evaluate the effects of poor sanitation on the health of the laboring class in Great Britain. Shortly thereafter, Lemuel Shalluck, one of the pioneers of public health in the United States, published a similar report on the health of workers in Massachusetts. For the next 50 years, however, there were practically no valuative studies of health or healthcare in the United States.

Concerns about quality in healthcare came to the forefront in 1910 and led to the landmark *Flexner Report*. Under the auspices of the Carnegie Foundation, Abraham Flexner, a young educator, collected and analyzed information on medical schools throughout the country. His report resulted in the closing of most of the country's substandard medical schools, the upgrading of others, and, in general, increased standardization of curricula.

Also in 1910, when the *Flexner Report* was receiving a great deal of public attention, a private, internal event occurred that was to eventually have far-reaching effects on the improvement of quality in healthcare. Dr. Ernest Codman, a Boston surgeon, while visiting professional colleagues in England, had a revelation in a hansom cab while returning to London from the Tuberculosis Sanitarium at Frimley. In a flash of insight, it struck Codman that the measurement of the end result is the tool by which all claims to surgical competence would be verified and the practice of surgery in hospitals standardized.

He became obsessed with the "end result idea," which, like many profound concepts, was quite simple. He described it as "merely the common-sense notion that every hospital should follow every patient it treats, long enough to determine whether or not the treatment has been successful, and then to inquire, if not, why not, with a view to preventing a similar failure in the future." To implement his idea Codman devised the "end result system," which he used in his small private hospital in Boston. This called for each patient to have a card on which were entered the symptoms, the diagnosis, the treatment plan, any complications that occurred, the diagnosis at discharge, and the results each year afterward until a definite determination of the outcome could be made.

Like many men whose ideas were before their time, Codman was not popular—or even accepted—by the established order; Massachusetts General Hospital, at which he had begun his surgical work, all but shunned him. Still, his pioneering work in quality improvement eventually gained recognition and in fact provided the basis of the 1918 Standardization Program of the American College of Surgeons. One example of Codman's theory put into practice was the Women's Hospital of New York, where a massive commitment to quality improvement—measured by evaluating end results, was described by Dr. George Ward in a paper presented at a meeting of the American College of Surgeons in 1923.

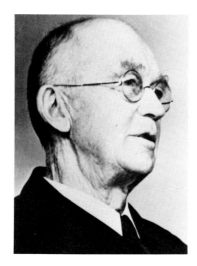

In addition to developing the standards to evaluate and accredit hospitals in the United States, Codman's lasting legacy is that he believed—and proved—that quality can be measured and determined. In a sense, Codman "demythologized" the pursuit of quality in medicine. While he admitted that some instances of care may be "like a priceless painting, incomparable in value," most care is "an ordinary commercial article whose quality can be standardized, and that can be produced more efficiently."

Thus the end result idea for Codman was the link between the science of medicine and the science of management. He was more a man of our time than of his because, while he was aware of the high calling of the medical profession, he recognized that the practice of medicine is also a business and that healthcare services compete in a marketplace: "Efficiency must acknowledge Truth and use it in a truthful way. It is the scientific use of science. I claim that the adoption of the End Result System by the hospitals of this country will at the same time render our work more scientific and our practice more efficient and honorable."

From the 1920s through most of the 1940s—through the years of recovery from World War I, the collapse of the economy in the 1930s, and entry into a second global war—little work was done in the area of assessing the quality of care in hospitals. In the 1940s interest was revived, and in 1948, Paul Lembcke—called "the father of the medical audit"—introduced his scientific method to evaluate the quality of healthcare services by analyzing the data from medical records. The classic work of Lembcke was followed by others examining the meaning of "quality of care." One of the most comprehensive of these analyses is found in the writings of Avedis Donabedian—who acknowledged the influence of Codman.

Accreditation as a Measure of Quality

In 1952 the Joint Commission on Accreditation of Hospitals was formed by several medical forces to provide a means to qualify the safe operation of hospitals. The organization, which later became the Joint Commission on Accreditation of Healthcare Organizations (JCAHO), is a powerful force in hospital management.

JCAHO was first considered a voluntary seal of approval that hospitals would seek out as an assurance to their

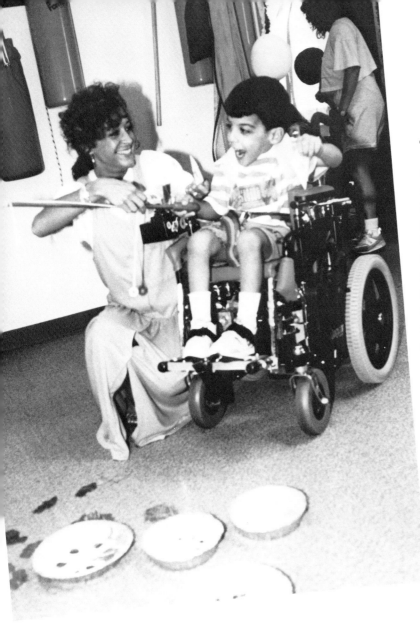

A speech pathologist works with a patient at the Institute for Child Development of Hackensack Medical Center, an internationally known evaluation and treatment program for children.
Courtesy, Hackensack Medical Center

Dr. William Silverman, Burdette Tomlin Memorial Hospital chief of pediatrics, relates one-on-one as he conducts a routine progress examination of one of his patients.
Photo by Craig Terry/Burdette Tomlin Memorial Hospital

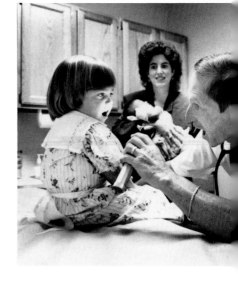

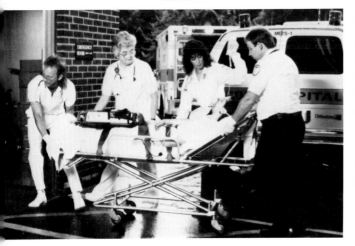

Leo Hayser, R.N., Rosaleen Fallon, R.N., MICU Coordinator Mary Lees, and MICU Supervisor Jeff Pack wheel a patient into Union Hospital Emergency Room, where life-saving decisions are just the beginning of a patient's total care.
Courtesy, Union Hospital

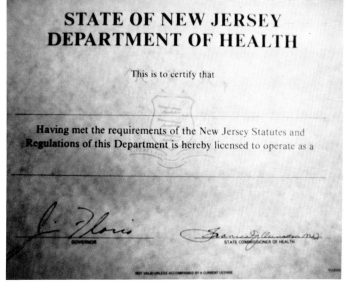

STATE OF NEW JERSEY
DEPARTMENT OF HEALTH

This is to certify that

Having met the requirements of the New Jersey Statutes and Regulations of this Department is hereby licensed to operate as a

GOVERNOR

STATE COMMISSIONER OF HEALTH

NOT VALID UNLESS ACCOMPANIED BY A CURRENT LICENSE

A basic of quality control is certification of healthcare professionals. As the industry changes, NJHA plays an important role in providing information and recommendations to the New Jersey Department of Health.

Courtesy, the New Jersey Department of Health

community that they met peer-established, objective national standards for measuring quality of hospitals. State government routinely conducted inspections in New Jersey, but other states across the country had minimal or no state inspection programs.

Over the years, JCAHO's accreditation has evolved from a voluntary program to one that is more or less mandatory. The federal government, for example, will reimburse Medicare and Medicaid patients for care given only in hospitals that are JCAHO accredited. Other third-party payors and managed care groups require that hospitals have JCAHO accreditation and meet other criteria regarding appropriateness of care and use of medical services.

As healthcare has grown in complexity, so too has the scope of the standards. In 1956, the JCAHO manual of standards for hospital accreditation was an eight-page document, and in 1992 it totaled 277 pages.

NJHA works closely with hospitals to prepare them for the JCAHO accreditation process, which occurs every three years. JCAHO changes its standards yearly in an ongoing process to keep pace with advances in medical technology and developments in healthcare management.

State Standards for Licensing

Since 1947, the state of New Jersey has licensed private hospitals under the auspices of various agencies and departments. In 1971, inspection duties mandated by the broad-sweeping Health Care Facilities Act came under the direction of the State Department of Health.

The state's inspections differ from JCAHO's in several ways. Historically, JCAHO has concentrated more on medical staff issues and the Department of Health more on facility issues. Additionally, when the state inspects a hospital, the failings of the hospital become part of public record—something consumers can examine and use to make determinations about where they would like to receive care. While JCAHO works closely with hospitals to pinpoint shortcomings and see that those insufficiencies are corrected, their inspection records are not available to the public.

New Jersey has endeavored to improve its statewide licensing of hospitals and upgrade the annual inspection program. Among numerous reforms, through various administrations and health commissioners, the Department of Health in 1986 undertook an ambitious licensure reform program to

revise the standards that had been in use some 20 years, and to develop new standards more reflective of current hospital operations. The process created to develop these new standards involved the participation of many healthcare professionals working in large and small hospitals throughout the state, as well as the New Jersey Hospital Association.

Some 32 areas of concern were addressed, ranging from anesthesia, discharge planning, medical staff, nurse staffing, and obstetrics to oncology, pediatrics, pharmacy, psychiatry, quality assurance, radiology, and social work. Groups of individuals working in the particular areas of concern were asked to suggest to the Department of Health what they thought were standards to measure quality of care in hospitals. Meeting after meeting was held and the exact wording of the standards reworked and refined. A statewide survey polled a larger number of healthcare professionals and incorporated their opinions into the standards. Standards were published in the *New Jersey Record* and commented upon by the public and NJHA before being refined again, the last becoming law in early 1992.

The new hospital standards were created to assure high quality care. As stated in the general provision of these regulations: "Components of quality care addressed by these rules and standards include access to care, continuity of care, comprehensiveness of care, coordination of services, humaneness of treatment, conservatism in intervention, safety of environment, professionalism of care givers, and participation in useful studies."

One of the important areas addressed in the new hospital standards for New Jersey is that of patient rights. Before adoption, the issue of patient rights was totally absent from previous standards. Now every patient has certain rights—to receive care, have access to information, refuse medication and treatment, and others—spelled out specifically and protected by law.

Moving Toward National Standards

How to measure quality in hospitals is an issue of continuing controversy. Many of the proposed standards were looked on as a wish list, very costly for hospitals to implement, and not necessarily valid or reliable measurements of quality. Many hospital industry leaders felt that other standards were too prescriptive and took away hospital management's prerogative to manage.

As an alternative to state licensing of hospitals, NJHA has introduced legislation to give *deemed* status to hospitals with JCAHO accreditation, something 42 states have done on a partial or full basis. Deemed status would mean that JCAHO has been granted authority, through legislation, to satisfy the New Jersey Department of Health's licensure requirements.

Some critics of deemed status cite the fact that

JCAHO inspects only every three years. However, many more professionals acknowledge that JCAHO standards are improved each year to incorporate the most current knowledge of equipment and identify areas where quality needs to be closely monitored, based on the operations of hospitals across the country. JCAHO's methodology and resources are much more sophisticated than any one state could possibly afford to assemble.

If deemed status were given to JCAHO-accredited New Jersey hospitals, the Department of Health would still have power to investigate any written complaint and conduct surveys for fire, life, and safety code violations. In addition, the Department of Health would receive the reports of JCAHO and be able to directly address the hospital with issues that are raised.

NJHA has taken the position that one reliable process is needed for evaluating the quality of patient care given in New Jersey hospitals. There are so many groups involved and each has its own standards for individual reasons—some of which have more to do with money than with care. Every request for information, whether it is a phone call or a chart review, places yet another administrative load on the administrative staffs of already burdened hospitals—and ultimately costs the healthcare consumer money.

Peer Review Organizations

The percentage of the nation's gross national product spent on healthcare had grown to more than 10 percent by 1983. To help bring the rapidly escalating costs of these programs under control, the federal government inaugurated the prospective payment system (PPS), which set a predetermined payment for Medicare patients, based on Diagnostic Related Groups (DRGs). In response to criticism that it was focusing exclusively on costs and realizing the incentives to offer fewer services under PPS, Congress set up a nationwide network of peer review organizations to ensure quality of care. Administered by the Health Care Financing Administration (HCFA), the Professional Standards Review Organizations (PSROs) were established to look at utilization first, then quality. They were comprised of local physicians whose responsibility was to review hospital admissions within their geographical area to determine whether hospitalization was medically necessary and if the treatment and length of stay were appropriate.

The PSROs were established to assure quality and to contain costs, two mandates that some feared were incompatible. In congressional testimony before the Subcommittee on Health of the House Ways and Means Committee in 1986, Jack Owen, former president of the New Jersey Hospital Association who was then the executive vice president of the American Hospital Association, said there was no evidence of deterioration in the quality of care given to Medicare beneficiaries under the new payment plan. Thus, measures that could contain costs—such as shorter hospital stays and hospital admissions only when medically necessary—could foster better, more appropriate and effi-

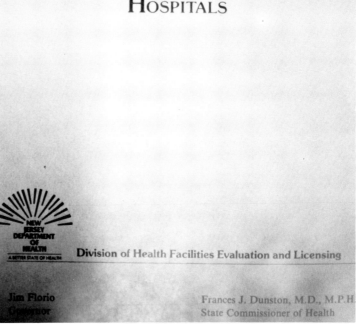

LICENSING STANDARDS
FOR
HOSPITALS

Division of Health Facilities Evaluation and Licensing

Jim Florio
Governor

Frances J. Dunston, M.D., M.P.H.
State Commissioner of Health

Rules and standards of licensing New Jersey hospitals address components of quality care, which include everything from safety and access to humaneness of treatment.
Courtesy, the New Jersey Department of Health

cient, as well as less costly care. The PSROs have been superseded by PROs, or Peer Review Organizations, which have broader responsibility for assuring quality of care, including the review of ambulatory patients.

Total Quality Management

Because of the escalating pressures to control costs and to ensure quality, and because of the difficulties with traditional quality assurance systems, healthcare organizations in the United States have begun to look at a new philosophy of "total quality management" (TQM), or "continuous quality improvement." Although the new approach may seem like a radical departure from traditional approaches, TQM actually is a natural outgrowth of the progression of quality assessment in healthcare over the last four decades, from medical audits, to peer review, to systematic quality assurance.

The concept of total quality management was developed in industry, first in Japan, and then, in the 1980s, in the United States. The principles were formulated by three Americans who are still considered the gurus of the quality field: W. Edwards Deming, Joseph M. Juran, and Philip B. Crosby. Although the three approaches have different emphases and components, they all center on understanding the complex processes in any industry, gathering data using reliable statistical methods, and using the information to build quality into the system, rather than focusing on inspection at the end.

Total quality management, as its name implies, encompasses the entire organization, from top to bottom and across all departments. It is a major premise of TQM that the organization's leadership be committed and that all employees be involved. TQM is not just another program—or separate function or department—but a new philosophy, a way of looking at quality and how it is continuously improved, that pervades the environment and culture of the organization.

What all TQM approaches have in common—and

with other total management experts—is the emphasis on statistical measurement, on total involvement of everyone in the organization, on the needs of the customers (anyone outside or inside the organization that receives a product or service), and on the process rather than the individual.

TQM views each person in an organization as part of interdependent processes; the overwhelming majority of failures in quality occur, not because of the fault of an individual, but because of the flaw in the process. Thus the importance of the system in production is a fundamental difference between modern quality management and traditional quality assurance programs that emphasize the performance of the individual. Since the organizational processes are responsible for more than 80 percent of quality problems, TQM theory discourages blaming individuals or exhorting them to work harder; instead they should be involved in analyzing production processes and systems. While the old assumption was that quality fails when people do the right things wrong, TQM theory asserts that it fails when people do the wrong things right.

Total Quality Management Applied to Healthcare—the National Demonstration Project

Since the basic concepts of TQM were developed first in manufacturing, they have a concrete and commercial flavor. Their proponents argued that their applications need not be restricted to industry. Quality experts insisted that TQM principles were a way to understand how productive activity occurs and could improve the quality in any organization, producing any kind of goods or services. Many in the healthcare field, however, were initially skeptical about whether the methods of industrial quality management could be applied to healthcare. The differences between the modern hospital and the modern factory seemed too profound. The inputs and outputs in a healthcare environment seemed too difficult to relate; hospitals often had not one but two lines of hierarchy, the administrative and the medical staff.

In 1987, the National Demonstration Project (NDP) showed that the principles of modern quality management could indeed be successfully transferred to hospitals and healthcare organizations. In this large-scale experiment, 21 experts in quality management from major American companies, universities, and consulting firms were matched with teams of representatives from 21 healthcare organizations, including hospitals, HMOs, and group practices. This landmark project showed that quality management held promise and poten-

tial for the healthcare field. Participants in the NDP said they "saw things in a new and different way." They concluded, among other things, that quality improvement tools can work in healthcare; that cross-functional teams are valuable in improving healthcare processes; that data useful for quality improvement abounds in healthcare; and that healthcare organizations may need a broader definition of quality.

The evidence of the NDP suggests that TQM—far from being just another program or interesting activity—will become an important basis for evaluating and delivering healthcare over the next decade. In recognition of this, the Joint Commission on Accreditation of Healthcare Organizations is making the transition to TQM principles in its standards for evaluating and accrediting hospitals. JCAHO launched the *Agenda for Change* in 1987 to refocus its standards to encourage the implementation of total quality management or continuous quality improvement.

New Jersey at the Forefront of Total Quality Management in Hospitals

NJHA has been a primary resource for New Jersey hospitals on information about TQM programs applied to healthcare and a model of leadership for other state associations. In 1991, with a $300,000 grant from Johnson & Johnson, NJHA's Health Research and Educational Trust (HRET) established the Center for the Advancement of Total Quality Management in Hospitals.

The center seeks to introduce every hospital in New Jersey to the principles of TQM and assist hospitals in initiating their own programs. To do this, the center offers information about TQM, including books, journal articles, and audiovisual materials; a selected bibliography published semiannually; a newsletter on quality

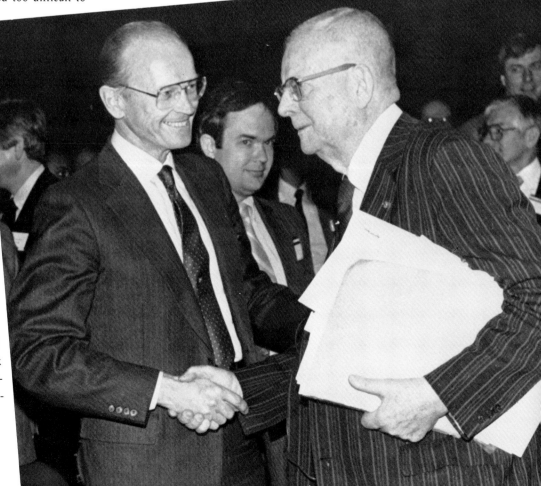

*d Motor Company sident Donald Peterson greets W. Edward ing, one of the quality rts whose concept of quality management is successfully being ied to the nation's thcare industry.
tesy, UPI/Bettmann*

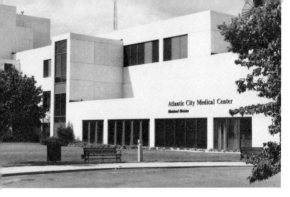

One of the first total quality management programs in New Jersey was conducted by Atlantic City Medical Center. Founded as a 10-bed hospital in a converted Victorian home in 1898, the medical center now is a 581-bed teaching facility that sees nearly 200,000 patients a year.
Courtesy, Atlantic City Medical Center

Continuous quality improvement concepts have been embraced by the staff of Saint Barnabas Medical Center in Livingston. Here, Kathy Koeller, a special testing technologist, monitors the dimensions and movement of the structures of the heart on a two-dimensional echocardiograph.
Courtesy, Saint Barnabas Medical Center

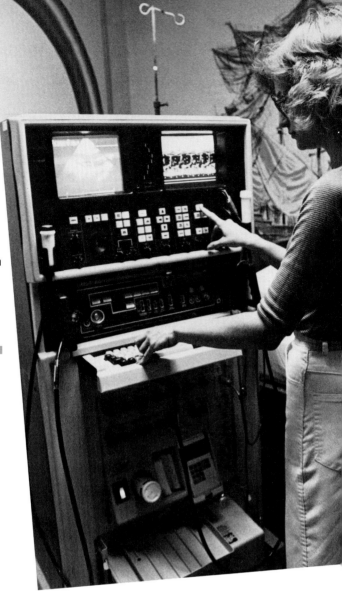

Quality care means addressing patients' concerns, as a child's stuffed panda receives medical attention from "Dr. Russ" at Our Lady of Lourdes Medical Center.
Courtesy, Our Lady of Lourdes Medical Center

Healthcare professionals and consumers are now being reached through extensive programs aimed at preventing injury and illness.
Photo by Mark E. Gibson

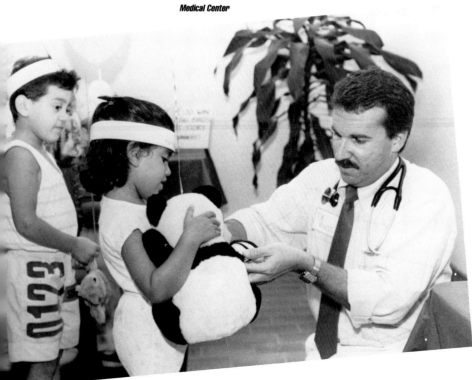

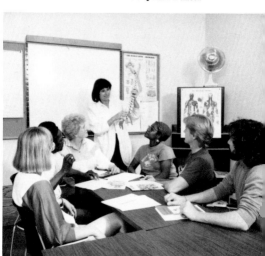

issues published especially for New Jersey hospitals; and a guide listing quality consultants and educational resources. In addition, the center sponsors conferences, seminars, and training forums on TQM for hospital staff and coordinates a speakers' bureau of local and national experts. The center also conducts research and provides specialized data services to hospitals. A major objective of the center is to build a statewide network in New Jersey among hospitals and between hospitals and industry.

As NJHA feels that different approaches meet the needs of different hospitals in different ways, it does not advocate one—for example, that of Deming, Juran, or Crosby—over another, but makes information available about a variety of theories, consultants, and organizations. To find out where New Jersey hospitals are now in TQM implementation, NJHA conducted a survey of how many hospitals had initiated modern quality management programs. The survey indicated that TQM is a new but growing phenomenon. Of the 60 hospitals that reported they have such programs, 70 percent reported that they have had them in place for a year or less; 15 percent have had programs for two to three years; and only 2 percent for four to five years. Interestingly, in contrast to the first projects of the NDP—which tended to focus on the business systems of hospitals—New Jersey hospitals apply quality principles to clinical quality improvement projects. The quality programs of many New Jersey hospitals also seem to successfully involve physicians on committees and work teams.

One of the first and most publicized hospital TQM programs in a New Jersey hospital was that of the Atlantic City Medical Center, which began its program in 1987. Like many hospitals that launch modern quality programs, Atlantic City started by surveying its patients and physicians to determine their attitudes and needs. The survey showed that while the medical center was highly respected for its technological capability and medical staff, it was not well regarded for its service elements, including cleanliness and employee attitudes.

In response, the Atlantic City Medical Center initiated a service improvement program called PACE, for Patients Are the Center of Everything. Training was held for all employees and management, and cross-departmental work teams were formed. Within a year, the teams implemented more than 200 improvements ranging from instituting valet parking to abolishing the requirement that respiratory therapists punch in on a time clock. The PACE program epitomized the effectiveness of the TQM approach; by collecting data, involving the entire organization, and looking at processes (rather than individuals), Atlantic City Medical Center achieved its goal of better service in hundreds of measurable ways.

The 15 hospitals that are members of the New Jersey branch of Voluntary Hospitals of America all have established quality management programs, initially implemented in response to VHA's interest. In 1987, VHA hired a national quality consulting firm to study the relationship among quality, cost, and market share in five clinical areas: surgical nervous system, surgical circulatory system, surgical joint/limb system, medical circulatory system, and medical pneumonia. The study, which covered nearly 62,000 patients discharged from all New Jersey hospitals in 1987, indicated that in four of the five areas (med-ical pneumonia was the exception), hospitals with higher quality had lower costs and greater market share.

Seeing the promise of quality management principles, VHA hospitals have become enthusiastic supporters of total quality principles and techniques. The management staff of Muhlenberg Regional Medical Center in Plainfield, for example, attended the Quality College of Philip Crosby Associates to learn how to set and monitor performance standards. Our Lady of Lourdes Medical Center in Camden, another VHA member hospital, has had a total quality program since October 1990, launched by its CEO and modeled on the theories of Deming; its seven initial project teams have spun off into 20, and ongoing educational efforts involve everyone in the organization. Monmouth Medical Center in Long Branch adopted the Crosby approach, and its successful TQM program is featured in many Crosby promotions, including videotapes, press kits, and brochures; the medical center credits quality management with reducing operating expenses by more than $2 million since March 1979.

The comprehensive quality improvement programs of Saint Barnabas Medical Center in Livingston uses an amalgam of the TQM theories, adapted to its own needs. While its official modern quality management program began in 1989, it was the natural outcome of its earlier quality assurance efforts; the more hospital staff studied patient surveys, the more they realized there were underlying process problems, and the more interested they became in TQM or continuous quality improvement concepts. Not only do Saint Barnabas's quality initiatives involve all staff and all departments, they also address both the clinical and nonclinical aspects of the hospital. Each month Saint Barnabas holds "QI Grand Rounds," seminars addressing quality improvement issues, and each spring the hospital stages a "QI Expo," highlighting the year's various projects.

The Future of Quality

The decade of the 1990s truly marks a turning point for healthcare in the United States. While not all players in New Jersey's healthcare crisis can agree on solutions, consensus is beginning to take shape around the need to work cooperatively to make a meaningful change. After controlling costs and increasing access, healthcare providers will face additional challenges and must look at incentives to prevent errors; the momentum will be toward quality.

New Jersey was an early believer in the premise that quality improvement and cost reduction go hand-in-hand, and the experiences in total quality management of many of its hospitals testify to this relationship. In the future, with the increasing pressures of the marketplace, the ultimate customers of healthcare—the patients and the payors—will no longer be willing to sacrifice one for the other. Quality concerns are moving to the forefront of healthcare issues, because of the recognition that quality, meaning both better service and less cost, will be the measure of success for healthcare institutions in the future. New Jersey hospitals, networking together through NJHA, are discovering the promise and potential—and excitement—that quality management ideas bring to healthcare.

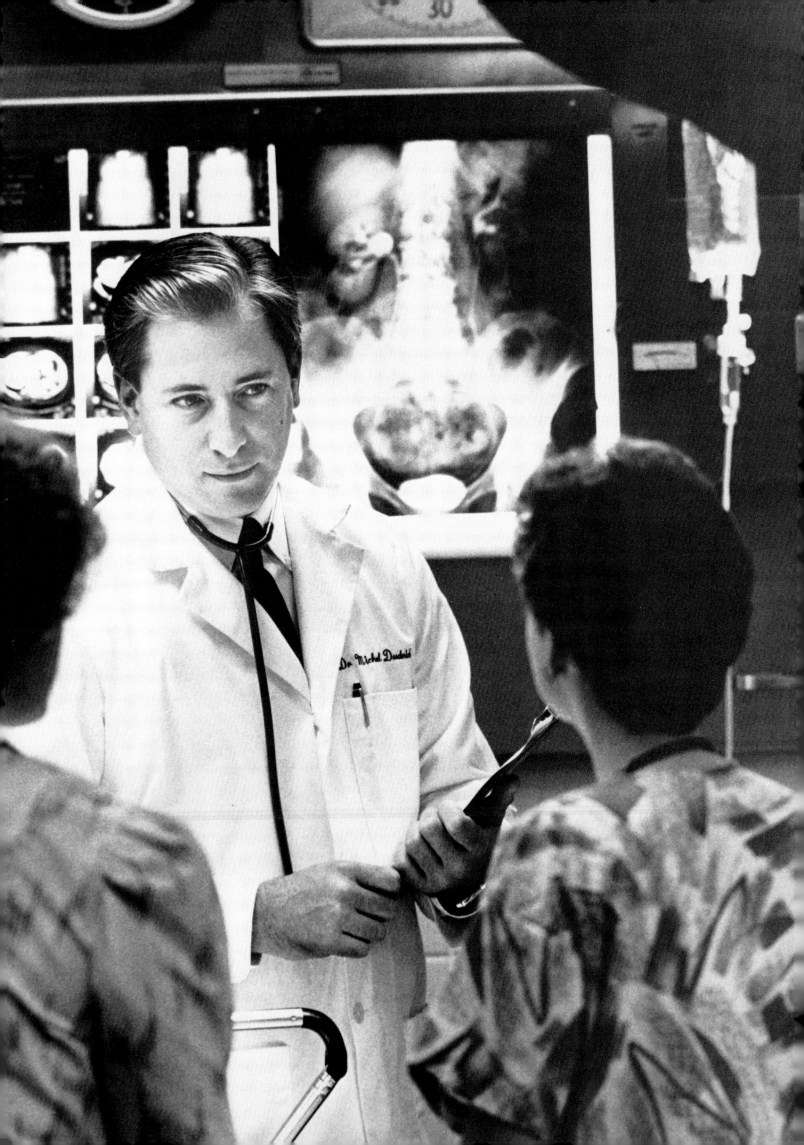

The healthcare professions and vocations are as old as the prehistory of humankind and as new as the technology of tomorrow. They are as diverse and varied as the fields of human endeavor, yet they have in common a unifying thread: contributing to the health and welfare of one's fellow beings.

Healthcare careers are demanding—and in demand. In New Jersey, more than 107,000 people are employed in hospitals, and the number of people—as well as the kinds of opportunities—is expanding rapidly. The health field offers the stability of employment as well as the excitement of being in the forefront of societal and technological change. There are also the rewards of being a part of a team and of doing work that matters. Healthcare careers offer the opportunity to "do well by doing good."

Although health careers in the late 20th century include more than 300 distinct professions and vocations in addition to that of physician and nurse, these two are certainly the oldest—and by centuries or millennia, not years or decades. Human beings cared for their sick long before written history. The examination of prehistoric bones and fossils indicates that primitive humans suffered from a variety of diseases and injuries. Archaeologists have discovered prehistoric skeletons with skillfully set fractures and skulls that show survival and healing after trephination, or surgical removal of disks of bone.

Prototypes of the two primary roles of physician and nurse existed in prehistory as the mother-nurse and physician-priest. The practice of nursing, which may have preceded the practice of the medicine man, gradually enlarged from the care and nourishment of infants and young children to the care of the sick, the aged, the infirm, and the disabled. As time progressed, it was increasingly recognized that love and caring alone were not sufficient to nurture health or overcome disease. Nursing came to be more dependent on two additional essential ingredients: skill and knowledge.

Similarly, the cures of the medicine man, or physician-priest, depended increasingly on the accumulated knowledge of folklore, incantations, and exorcisms—which became too complex to be understood by ordinary tribesmen. Certain chosen individuals who had special insight and training became the guardians and interpreters of the magical, healing lore for the benefit of the tribe. These men, and sometimes women, might have lived through some mystical experience, spent long periods alone in

CHAPTER 7

HEALTHCARE CAREERS

The Healing Arts and Sciences

Physician director of the Burdette Tomlin Memorial Hospital emergency services department, Michael Dudnick, confers with two of the specially trained nurses on staff.
Photo by Craig Terry/Burdette Tomlin Memorial Hospital

the wilderness, or recovered from critical illness or injury.

It is possible that the mother-nurse and the physician-priest were at first united but eventually divided into two practitioners of the healing art—the care giver and the cure giver. Or, even if the mother-nurse emerged first, as the caste of medicine men developed, the "wise women" of the tribe became a class of practitioners associated with them, applying treatments, administering medicinal plants, and dressing wounds.

The interdependence and interrelationship of these two primary healing roles is evident throughout history. In some periods, such as the Hippocratic era in the ancient world, the rational medicine of the physician functioned without nursing, whereas at other times, in the Middle Ages for example, nursing was practiced without theoretical medicine. Still, from the Stone Age until the 20th century, the two prototypical professions of nurse and physician developed, complementing and sometimes competing with the other.

Nursing—which has been called "the oldest of the arts and the youngest of the professions"—was transformed by Florence Nightingale in the mid-1800s. Although she did not establish nursing, she established nursing as a profession, laying the foundation for nursing principles and education not only in her native Britain, but in the world.

Most of the hundreds of healthcare careers available today evolved from either the practice of nursing or the practice of medicine. From its beginnings, nursing was a form of community service—the care and protection of members of the family group or tribe. The clinical and technical specialties emerged from the physician's role, with the advances in medical theory and technology.

As more sophisticated civilizations developed, the care of the sick expanded to include concern for other causes of suffering. Methods for dealing with problems such as poverty, prevention of disease, and any type of dependency added a social dimension to nursing. From an historical perspective, the nurse and the social worker are one. Only relatively recently did a separate profession emerge to deal specifically with the social ills of society.

The Present Diversity of Healthcare Careers

Hundreds of separate professions and vocations in healthcare encompass all fields of human endeavor and suit any individual talents or abilities. Most have evolved from the role of the physician, with the advancing medical technology, or from the role of the nurse, with the increasing professionalism. Some are medical adaptations or specializations of other professions, such as librarians, public relations professionals, accountants, or administrators. For an overview, these hundreds of job titles can be classified

into five categories, with subcategories in each:
- Direct care, including careers in medical, nursing, dental, and mental health subcategories
- Diagnostic, including careers in radiology, medical laboratories, diagnostic equipment, optical, and audiology/speech pathology
- Therapeutic/rehabilitative, including careers in physical, corrective, occupational, respiratory, recreational, music, dance, and art therapy, as well as orthotics and prosthetics, dietetics, and pharmacy
- Community/public health, including careers in statistics, sanitation, environmental issues, health education and communication, and home health services
- Support services, including careers in engineering, administration, personnel or human resources, accounting, payroll, purchasing, public relations, medical records, medical libraries, housekeeping, and maintenance

Careers in direct care, which include the traditional professions, are by far the largest number. To give some idea of the number and variety of careers in this category, direct care includes all kinds of physicians—doctors of medicine (who may have specialized in anything from cardiac surgery, dermatology, family practice, geriatrics, histology, or internal medicine to obstetrics, oncology, ophthalmology, neurology, pathology, pediatrics, radiology, or urology), as well as doctors of osteopathy, doctors of chiropractic, and doctors of podiatry. Nursing positions include professional, or registered nurses (R.N.s), nurse practitioners, licensed practical nurses (L.P.N.s), and licensed vocational nurses (L.V.N.s). Dentists may be doctors of dental surgery (D.D.S.s) or doctors of dental medicine (D.D.M.s) and may specialize in orthodontics, periodontics, or dentistry for children, the elderly, or the handicapped.

Direct care occupations encompass physician, medical, nursing, and dental assistants; nursing and geriatric aides; dental hygienists; and emergency medical technicians. Careers in the mental health field include psychiatrists (M.D.s), clinical psychologists (Ph.D.s), mental health technicians, orderlies, and psychiatric aides. In addition to working in hospitals, individuals in direct healthcare occupations also work in private practices, health maintenance organizations (HMOs), nursing homes, rehabilitation centers, state institutions, clinics, community emergency centers, and patients' homes.

Support services are an interesting category of careers, as they illustrate how so many professions today can be tailored to the healthcare field. University-based degree

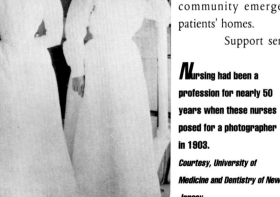

Nursing had been a profession for nearly 50 years when these nurses posed for a photographer in 1903.

Courtesy, University of Medicine and Dentistry of New Jersey

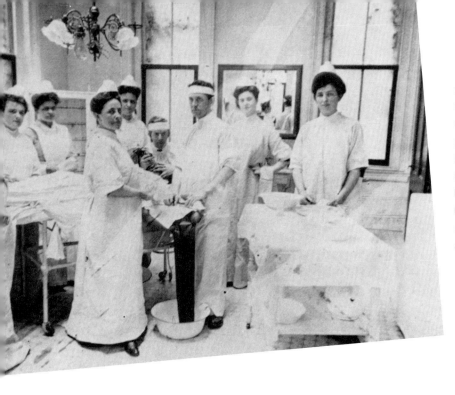

*T*he countless specialties of today had not yet evolved in the early 1900s, when surgery was performed with numerous nurses and assistants in attendance at St. Joseph's Hospital and Medical Center.
Courtesy, St. Joseph's Hospital and Medical Center

*A*t the Kessler Institute for Rehabilitation, clients simulate their jobs to build strength and endurance in preparation for returning to work. Plumber Mark Calabrese learns proper body mechanics under the watchful eye of administrative director Carol Harnett and another client, Vinston King.
Photo by Sharon Guynup/Kessler Institute for Rehabilitation

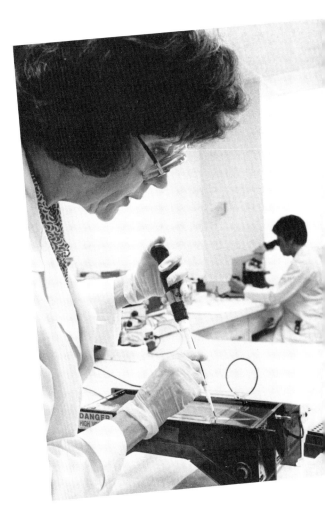

*P*recise analyses are performed by Janeen Dougherty, molecular pathology technician at the Institute for Molecular Diagnostics and Pathology at St. Peter's Medical Center, New Brunswick, and (background) Mona Crawford, cytology supervisor.
Courtesy, St. Peter's Medical Center

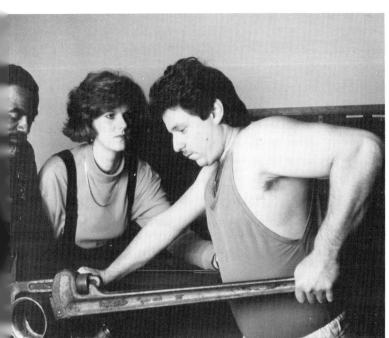

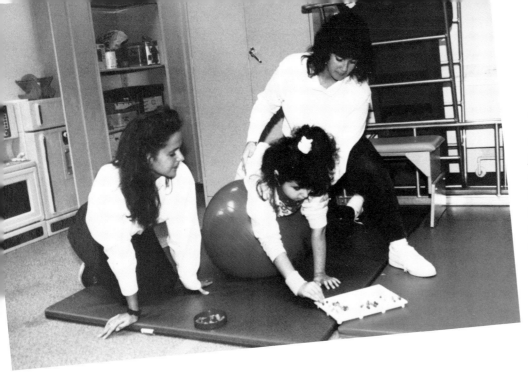

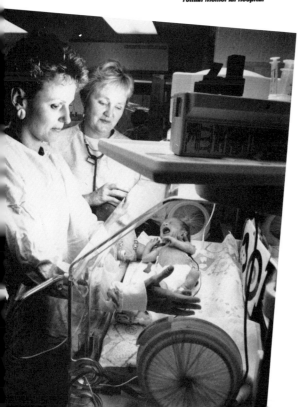

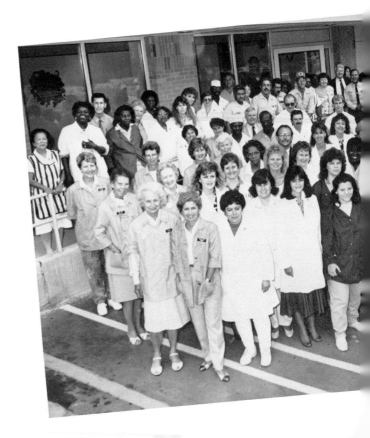

programs in hospital administration have existed since the 1920s. Medical engineers apply engineering principles to everything from developing computer-based models of blood composition to designing adaptive rehabilitation equipment. Hospital communications professionals apply public relations, marketing, and advertising expertise to meet the goals of a nonprofit service organization.

Medical—or health services or healthcare—libraries are an excellent example of specialized support service centers. Tremendous advances in medical knowledge and computer technology during the last two decades have transformed health services libraries into invaluable, state-of-the-art resource centers. In a recent study, 97 percent of the physicians surveyed said that the information provided by the hospital library contributed to better informed clinical care, and 80 percent said they actually handled some aspect of the care of their patients differently as a result of information provided by the library. Healthcare librarians offer a wide range of services to physicians, to other health professionals—dentists, nurses, pharmacists, and veterinarians—and to researchers, medical writers, medical illustrators, lawyers, and hospital administrators. Healthcare librarians work not only in hospitals, but in medical, dental, nursing, and veterinary schools, as well as in pharmaceutical companies, research facilities, government agencies, and a variety of foundations and associations. NJHA pioneered the establishment of healthcare management libraries within state hospital associations. Of the four states that have such libraries, the NJHA library, located at the Center for Health Affairs in Princeton and under the direction of the Health Research and Educational Trust of New Jersey, was the first—and remains the largest.

Education for Healthcare Careers

The education required for healthcare careers can range from perhaps 10 years of higher education for a highly specialized physician to a high school diploma for an entry-level aide or support services worker. Many healthcare occupations such as medical technicians, dental hygienists, practical nurses, and clerical workers require specialized vocational training or an associate's degree. Most professional positions—professional nurses, social workers, business administrators, laboratory technologists—require a bachelor's degree, and many require a specialized master's degree.

In New Jersey, physicians as well as a wide variety of health professionals are trained at the University of Medicine and Dentistry of New Jersey (UMDNJ). The largest freestanding health-sciences university in the United States, UMDNJ has three medical schools: the New Jersey Medical School (Newark campus); Rutgers Medical School (with two campuses, Piscataway and the school's clinical campus at Cooper Hospital/University Medical Center in Camden); and the New Jersey School of

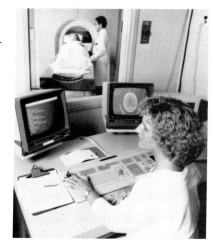

Osteopathic Medicine (Piscataway and the school's clinical campus at Kennedy Memorial Hospitals–University Medical Center). UMDNJ is unique as the only health-sciences institution in the country that educates D.O. (doctors of osteopathy) students together with M.D. students. For the first two years of basic study, students at the School of Osteopathic Medicine share classes and facilities with students at the Rutgers Medical School. In addition to the three medical schools, UMDNJ consists of the New Jersey Dental School, the Graduate School of Biomedical Sciences, and the Schools of Health-Related Professions, all located in Newark.

New Jersey offers many varied opportunities for individuals who want to prepare for nursing careers. Eleven colleges and universities in New Jersey offer four-year baccalaureate nursing programs, 13 community colleges offer two-year associate degree programs in nursing, and 17 New Jersey hospitals operate nursing schools with diploma programs. Graduates of the baccalaureate, associate, and diploma programs are eligible to take the licensure examination to practice as a registered nurse (R.N.). In addition, 21 institutions provide a one-year basic nursing skills program that enables graduates to take the licensing examination to become a licensed practical nurse (L.P.N.). In addition to vocational and technical schools, three New Jersey hospitals—Bergen Pines County Hospital, Hunterdon Medical Center, and Holy Name Hospital—offer L.P.N. programs. Rutgers, the State University, offers four-year nursing programs on both its New Brunswick and Camden campuses and is also the primary institution in New Jersey for undergraduate and graduate degrees in related professions such as social work, library science, business administration, and laboratory technology. Most of these degree programs can be tailored for individuals planning to specialize and apply their chosen profession in the healthcare field.

To address the educational issues that arise from the rapid changes occurring in all healthcare professions, NJHA established a Council on Education in 1990. The council, one of the first such initiatives of any state hospital association in the country, brings together expert representatives from hospitals and educational institutions to identify issues and develop initiatives in those areas requiring action. The council develops NJHA positions on healthcare education issues for recommendations to professional boards,

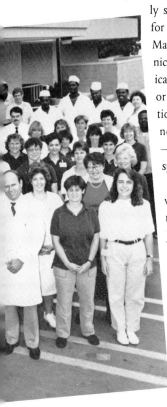

government agencies, and the legislature. Currently, one of the significant issues being studied by NJHA is graduate medical education, especially resource allocation and reimbursement policies in New Jersey.

In addition to educational qualifications, licensing, registration, or certification may also be required for healthcare professionals to practice in New Jersey. Physicians and physician assistants are licensed by the Board of Medical Examiners. Nurses—including nurse practitioners, registered nurses, and practical nurses—are licensed by the Board of Nursing. In addition, pharmacists and pharmacy technicians are licensed by the Board of Pharmacy; radiation therapy and nuclear medicine technologists by the Radiology Technology Board/Board of Examiners; physical therapists by the Board of Physical Therapy; and respiratory therapists and respiratory therapy technicians by the Board of Respiratory Care. Medical records administrators and technicians must receive a passing score on a credentialing examination, while occupational therapists may be certified, although there are no formal credentialing requirements. As healthcare occupations change rapidly—and as there are different licensing boards and certifying authorities for different fields—NJHA plays an important role as a clearinghouse for information and a forum for the study and discussion of credentialing issues.

Meeting the Demand for Healthcare Personnel

Healthcare professions and vocations are attractive because they are generally personally rewarding, socially respected, well-paying, and full of opportunities for advancement. Although many individuals enter careers in health, problems in supply and demand do exist—especially in some job categories and geographical areas, and especially for hospitals, compared to other healthcare employers. As the ranks of rural and inner-city physicians have thinned, physician assistants (P.A.s), who first emerged in the 1960s, have been in great demand. P.A.s work under an M.D.'s supervision and have the authority to order and interpret laboratory tests, diagnose illnesses, suture wounds, and in some states, prescribe medicines. Although the original role of the P.A. was to assist primary care physicians in the "underserved" geographical areas, since the 1970s they have increasingly assumed roles in hospital-based healthcare. NJHA, realizing that P.A.s have much to offer hospitals in terms of care delivery, supported the efforts of the Board of Medical Examiners to establish two-year pilot programs to study the use of P.A.s in certain supervised settings. The Physician Assistant Licensing Act was passed in June 1992.

Nurse practitioners and clinical nurse specialists have also gained increased responsibility and autonomy in recent years. These highly trained professionals can be key to the provision of primary care and can be effectively used in managed care, outpatient, clinic, and other ambulatory services affiliated with hospitals and the local community. NJHA felt that giving nurse practitioners and certified nurse specialists the authority to prescribe medications would provide even greater access to healthcare in New Jersey.

Collaborating with the New Jersey State Nurses Association, the Organization of Nurse Executives, and the New Jersey League of Nurses, NJHA facilitated the passage of state legislation granting these professionals certain prescriptive authority. Also, NJHA assisted a special task force of the State Board of Nursing to develop the regulations governing the prescriptive powers of nurse practitioners and clinical nurse specialists.

Although shortages in any healthcare profession can cause critical problems for hospitals, shortages in nursing have traditionally been the most pervasive and troublesome. NJHA has been a leader—and a model in the nation—for its innovative initiatives in addressing shortages in the healthcare professions, especially in nursing. In 1988, NJHA launched the Nursing Resource Center, the first ever in New Jersey and one of the first in the country. A year later, the center was expanded to address the critical shortage in other health professions. The purpose of the Nursing and Allied Health Resource Center is to encourage qualified individuals to pursue careers in nursing and health-related fields. By calling the center's two toll-free telephone numbers, 1-800-356-NURSE and 1-800-66-ALLIED, individuals may receive personalized information on educational programs in New Jersey; financial aid, scholarships, and tuition reimbursement; high school prerequisites; licensure requirements and dates of licensure examinations; employment opportunities, including a list of New Jersey hospitals; salary ranges; and professional associations and organizations. Monthly listings of the names and addresses of callers are sent to New Jersey nursing programs and hospitals for follow-up. The computerized logging and tracking system of the Nursing and Allied Health Resource Center also allows comprehensive data to be collected and analyzed for planning and marketing.

With its Resource Center, NJHA quickly became recognized as the primary clearinghouse for information about healthcare occupations in New Jersey, not only among hospitals but among state and voluntary associations as well. The Medical Society of New Jersey has endorsed NJHA's Resource Center as the "informational clearinghouse and referral source for individuals interested in nursing and allied health professions." The Health Occupations Students of America/New Jersey works with the center to increase the number of young people participating in its organization. The New Jersey Department of Health's Nursing Advisory Committee has formally sanctioned, in its bylaws, collaborative activity with the Resource Center to ensure "valid information regarding the education and practice of nursing." The Department of Higher Education has requested NJHA's participation on its Advisory Committee on Allied Health Employment Issues. The Department of Labor is working with the Resource Center to help recently unemployed workers—especially those in fields affected by recession or new employment trends—to seek jobs in New Jersey hospitals or pursue professional healthcare careers. The Resource Center continues to work closely with the New Jersey State Nurses Association, the Organization of Nurse Executives,

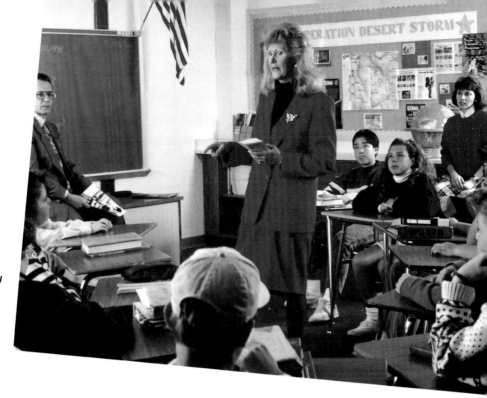

*N*JHA's community outreach programs encourage students to consider the growing occupational needs of the healthcare industry.
Courtesy, New Jersey Hospital Association

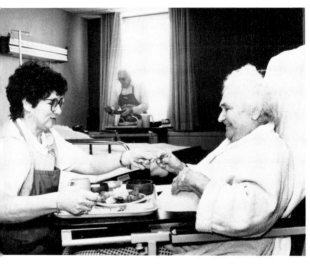

*V*olunteer coordinator for the Silver Spoons program at Burdette Tomlin Memorial Hospital, Natalie Milcarsky assists a patient while Bart Sereni prepares a tray.
Photo by Craig Terry/Burdette Tomlin Memorial Hospital

*E*mbraced by registered nurse and former Miss America Kaye Lani Ray Rafko, candy stripers are off to a good start as they help NJHA's Nursing and Allied Health Resource Center promote healthcare careers.
Courtesy, New Jersey Hospital Association

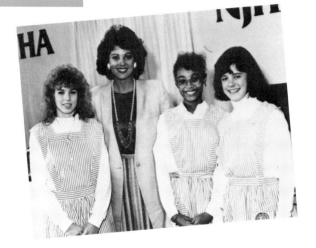

*T*oday's healthcare industry provides a wide variety of career opportunities. Here, Chief Perfusionist Peter Mueller monitors equipment at Jersey Shore Medical Center Heart Institution.
Courtesy, Jersey Shore Medical Center

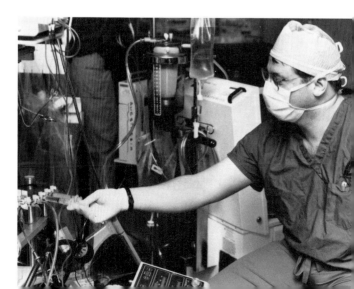

and the New Jersey League of Nurses.

To encourage New Jerseyans to call the Resource Center—and to increase the general public's awareness of the opportunities in healthcare—NJHA launched a nationally recognized, award-winning marketing campaign in 1988. Based on the theme "The Rewards of a Life's Work," the campaign featured television and radio public service announcements, informational videotapes, brochures, posters, billboard advertisements throughout the state, and inserts in national magazines. Serving as a model for other states, the marketing campaign package was purchased by several other state hospital associations.

Largely because of the success of the campaign, which directed people to the center's toll-free numbers, NJHA's Resource Center has received more than 10,000 inquiries since it began in 1988. Sixty-three percent of respondents to a follow-up survey applied to or enrolled in a nursing or allied health program or have pursued employment in a hospital or healthcare facility. The Hospital Nursing Services Survey, published annually by NJHA, documents the progress New Jersey has made in addressing the nursing shortage. The vacancy rate for professional nurses—which was an alarming 17 percent in 1988—has dropped to 6.6 percent, well below the national average. Vacancy rates in other health professions have fallen significantly, if not as dramatically.

The Adopt-A-School Program

Callers to the Resource Center, however, fall primarily into the 25- to 40-year-old age group. "The Reward's of a Life's Work" marketing campaign, while successful in targeting adults, did not reach New Jersey's youth. To provide a stimulus to young people, NJHA formed a grassroots effort to forge relationships between New Jersey hospitals and their neighborhood schools. Through this innovative effort, called the Adopt-A-School program, high school students are introduced to information about healthcare careers and meet professionals who can serve as role models. Guidance counselors, teachers, and parents are also targeted audiences.

Among the state's hospitals that have strong and varied Adopt-a-School programs, Bayshore Community Hospital in Holmdel, Camden County Health Services Center, and Rahway Hospital offer a pre-health careers course, taught by members of their hospital staffs. Several hospitals offer mentorship programs to students from their adopted schools: Camden County Health Services Center, Community Medical Center in Toms River (Toms River High School North), Newark Beth Israel Medical Center (Maple High School), Rahway Hospital (Rahway High School), St Clares*Riverside (Morris Catholic High School), and Union Hospital (Union High School and Abraham Clark High School). Hackensack Medical Center employs students who are not college bound, and Newark Beth Israel Medical Center offers summer employment as well as scholarships for students choosing to enter healthcare fields. Many other hospitals have similar programs.

Health careers fairs are especially popular: Helene Fuld Medical Center in Trenton, The Memorial Hospital of Salem County, Memorial Hospital of Burlington County, The Mercer Medical Center, Monmouth Medical Center, Muhlenberg Regional Medical Center in Plainfield, Overlook Hospital in Summit, St. Joseph's Hospital and Medical Center in Paterson, and St. Peter's Hospital in New Brunswick are among the hospitals in all parts of the state that offer career fairs for students from their adopted high schools.

Reaching the Older Healthcare Worker

As New Jersey's major companies experience work force reductions, the healthcare industry continues to grow. This pool of older, experienced workers creates another excellent source of health career recruits. Through NJHA initiatives, the New Jersey Department of Labor—when responding to a company that is reducing its work force—now provides information about healthcare employment opportunities to the individuals affected by layoffs. Persons referred to the Nursing and Allied Health Resource Center receive personalized counseling concerning healthcare occupations, ranging from nontechnical, nonprofessional positions in New Jersey's hospitals to professional and highly skilled roles requiring advanced education. The Resource Center can also directly link prospective employees with hospital personnel departments or prospective students with New Jersey schools. In addition to assisting the mature individual making a career change, the statistical profiles of these callers provide invaluable data to NJHA in planning to meet the needs of the ever-increasing number of older, nontraditional students and employees.

The Nursing Incentive Reimbursement Awards

Although NJHA's Nursing and Allied Health Resource Center has made a dramatic difference, an increased demand for nurses is predicted for New Jersey as well as throughout the country. Since it is difficult for the supply of professional nurses to equal the demand, NJHA works with hospitals to address their nursing shortages in other innovative ways. NJHA provided leadership and assistance to hospitals seeking grants from the New Jersey Department of Health under the Nursing Incentive Reimbursement Awards (NIRA) program. An independent panel selected 23 New Jersey hospitals to receive the grants, which ranged from $150,000 to $500,000, to initiate creative projects to address the nursing shortage—from either a demand-side or a supply-side perspective.

Despite the diversity of their approaches, the hospitals' projects fell into four categories. Several hospitals proposed projects that restructured the way nursing services are delivered. For example, Our Lady of Lourdes Medical Center implemented a practice model for nurses, patterned after physician group practice, in which nurses are organized into "nurse associate practices," of a nursing case manager, an R.N., an L.P.N., and a nurse's aide. At St. Francis Medical Center and at Hackensack Medical Center, an R.N. and an

L.P.N. or nurse's assistant work together as a team. John F. Kennedy Medical Center in Edison organized pilot units of two teams, each consisting of an R.N., an L.P.N., and a nurse's aide. At Riverview Medical Center, case managers were made responsible for following selected high-risk patients. The Medical Center of Ocean County changed nursing care from a task-oriented to a modular, team approach to conserve time and to allow R.N.s to become more involved in direct care.

Another broad category of projects implemented by hospitals receiving NIRA grants were initiatives that restructured the working environment for nurses. Newark Beth Israel Medical Center added a service attendant, reporting to nursing, to each pilot unit to take responsibility for many of the housekeeping, dietetic, and transporting services. Hunterdon Medical Center and Morristown Memorial Hospital developed "shared governance" projects, in which nurses were given greater autonomy and responsibility.

Computer projects were popular choices for NIRA projects; 15 of the 23 participating hospitals implemented new bedside or unit-base computer systems to assist nurses. The eight New Jersey hospitals that implemented such systems in 1990 were national pioneers: Community Medical Center in Toms River, Dover General Hospital and Medical Center, Hunterdon Medical Center, Memorial Hospital of Burlington County, Our Lady of Lourdes Medical Center, Shore Memorial Hospital, Southern Ocean County Hospital, and St. Francis Medical Center. As recently as 1989, fewer than 50 hospitals in the entire United States had bedside computer systems.

*F*rom coordination and dispatch to piloting and mechanical upkeep, support personnel are needed in all fields of healthcare transportation. *Courtesy, St. Joseph's Hospital and Medical Center*

Four New Jersey hospitals initiated education projects, another category into which the NIRA awards fell. Community Medical Center prepared videotapes, book-

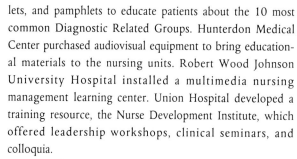

lets, and pamphlets to educate patients about the 10 most common Diagnostic Related Groups. Hunterdon Medical Center purchased audiovisual equipment to bring educational materials to the nursing units. Robert Wood Johnson University Hospital installed a multimedia nursing management learning center. Union Hospital developed a training resource, the Nurse Development Institute, which offered leadership workshops, clinical seminars, and colloquia.

The imaginative projects spurred by the NIRA grants, awarded in 1989 and 1990, have been evaluated by the Health Research Program of New York University, to determine the long-term results and benefits. This evaluative information is intended to support the diffusion of successful innovations to other hospitals, throughout the country as well as in New Jersey.

The Future of Healthcare Careers

In 1950, the healthcare industry was the nation's fifth leading employer; today it ranks as the second leading industry. The reasons the tremendous expansion came about were the increased population, longer life spans, advances in technology, and the public's demand for quality healthcare. In 1986, 7.6 million workers were employed in the healthcare industry across the nation; the projection for 2000 is 10.8 million healthcare workers. One out of every six new jobs will be in the health field.

As the nation's most urban and densely populated state—with a median-age elderly population second only to Florida—New Jersey must meet the rapidly growing needs for trained health workers and professionals before most other states. Even for the immediate future, projections of New Jersey's healthcare personnel needs in 1995 are striking. The demand for nurses will increase by almost 50 percent, or 22,600 positions; for physical therapists, now the most sought-after healthcare profession after nursing, by 41 percent; for respiratory therapists, 40 percent; for dental hygienists, 39 percent. The need for radiography technologists will increase by 36 percent; for dietitians, 29 percent; and for paramedics, 24 percent. These statistics compare with a projected increase in demand for nonhealth fields by 1995 of only 16 percent.

Besides the rapid growth in numbers and demand, many other developing trends will characterize healthcare careers in the years to come: the role of women in the work force, the aging of the population, competition and the quest for excellence, and changing approaches to the delivery of health services. With its creative initiatives, New Jersey has seen the future—and has pioneered innovative ways to supply the demand for highly qualified and motivated individuals in the healing arts and sciences.

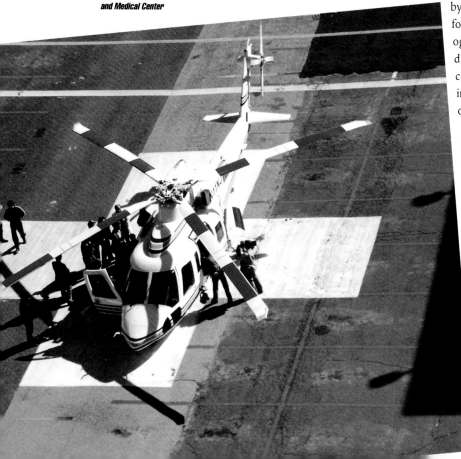

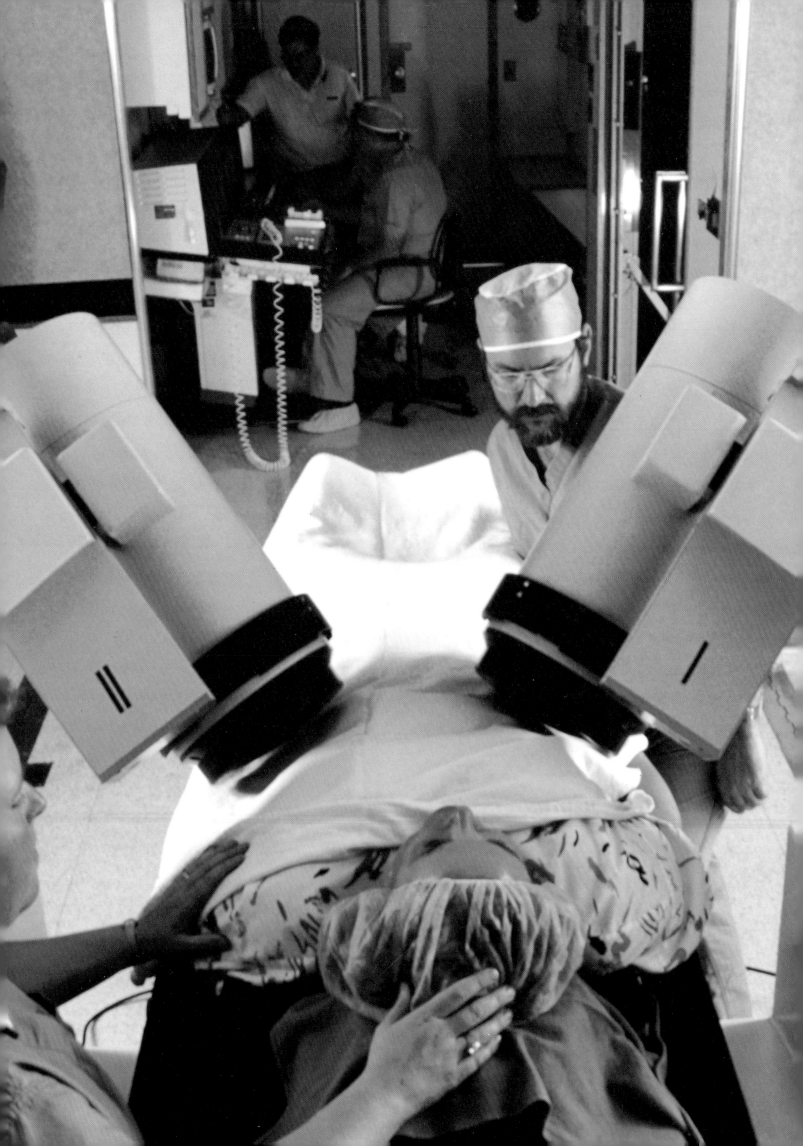

*A*s medical technology continues to evolve at lightening speed, professionals must be trained to perform delicate procedures, such as lithotripsy, a noninvasive procedure in which electro-hydraulic shock waves are used primarily to pulverize kidney stones.
Photo by Tom Raymond/Medichrome

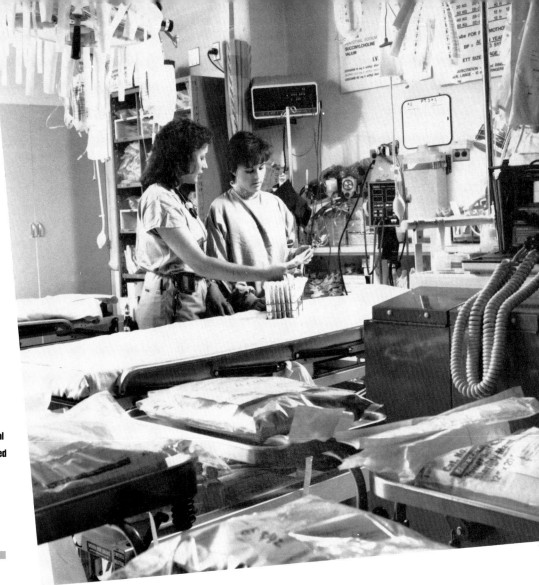

*J*ust as yesterday's equipment is obsolete, today's advanced medical practices will be replaced by even more effective procedures tomorrow.
Courtesy, Cooper Hospital/University Medical Center

*T*he Cardiac Rehabilitation Program at Pascack Valley Hospital provides a medically supervised exercise program that assists those diagnosed with, or at risk of developing, heart disease.
Courtesy, Pascack Valley Hospital

A hospital pharmacist measures the appropriate medication ordered for a patient—an integral part of hospital care.
Photo by John Greim/Medichrome

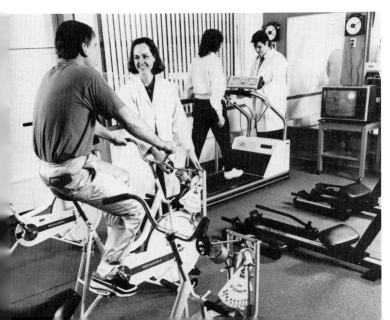

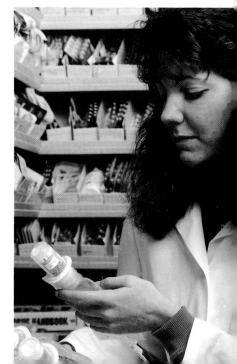

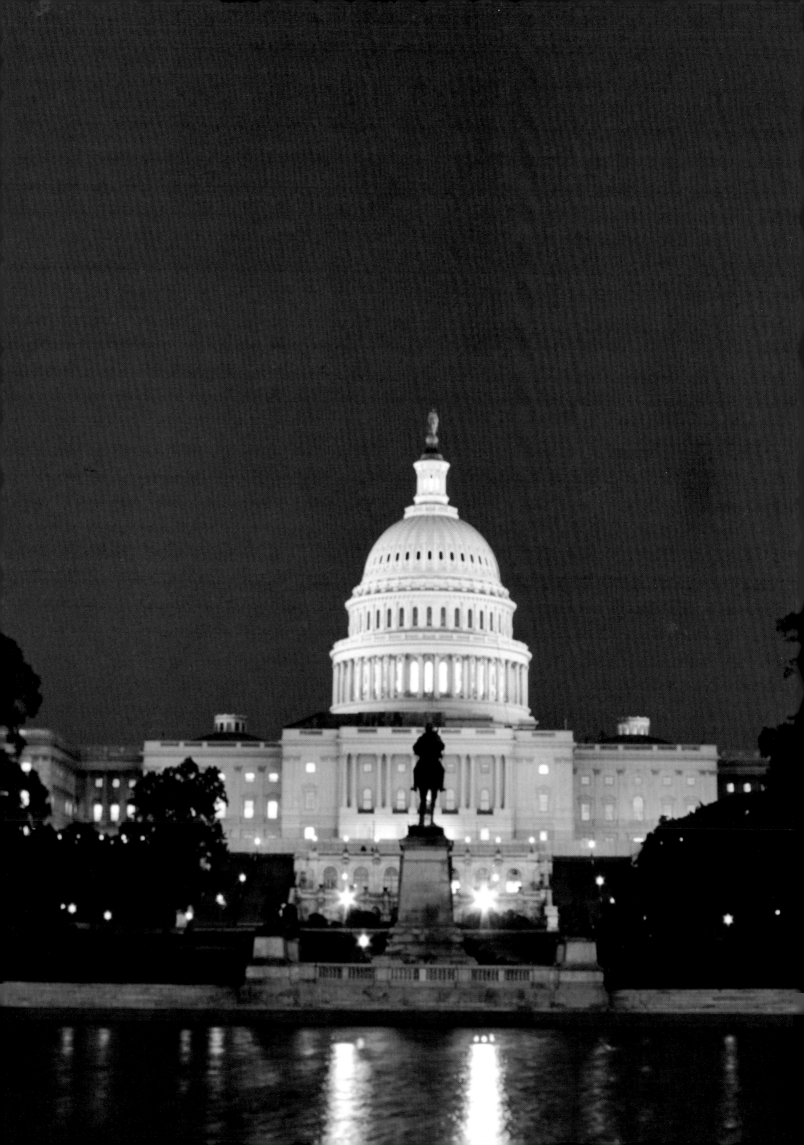

The governance and management of American hospitals, including those in New Jersey, have reflected the social order and sources of authority throughout history. The earliest hospitals were governed by pious and paternalistic trustees, who sought to impose a moral order on the operation of the institutions—as well as upon their inmates. At the beginning of the 20th century, with society's new respect for science and technology, authority in hospitals shifted from lay trustees to physicians. By midcentury, as the operation of hospitals became more complex and involved more "outsiders," such as legislators, government officials, and third-party payors, hospital administrators became more powerful. For a variety of historical reasons, these three centers of authority—trustees, physicians, and administrators—remain essential but distinct entities in the governing and management of today's hospitals.

The earliest American hospitals provided a home and surrogate family for individuals who were not only ill, but socially and economically dependent. The emphasis was not on medical cure, but upon care and meeting basic needs for food, clothing, and shelter. Trustees—as embodiments of the community's values and stewards of its resources—founded these institutions and oversaw every aspect of their operation.

For the lay trustees, the only appropriate model for these institutions was the family. A superintendent or steward appointed by the trustees as their representative was the patriarchal head of the household, responsible for purchasing necessities and disciplining both patients and house staff. His wife often served as the matron, in charge of cooking, cleaning, laundry, and supervision of the women's wards. The superintendent and his wife and children lived at the hospital and ate meals with the staff. Not surprisingly, the qualities the trustees sought in a superintendent were not hospital experience or medical training but prudence, piety, and frugality.

Regulations for staff and patients alike were aimed at controlling behavior. House staff, nurses, and domestics, as well as patients, needed a pass to leave the grounds. Discipline was complicated by the fact that most patients were ambulatory; in most hospitals authorities withheld the patients' clothes to control their coming and going. Punishment was administered in the form of cold showers, bread-and-water diets, and isolation. Nevertheless, despite the efforts of the hospital "parents," truancy

HOSPITAL GOVERNANCE AND MANAGEMENT

Changing Order and Unchanging Mission

*H*ealthcare decisions made in the New Jersey legislature directly affect other states and the future of national reform.
Photo by Mark E. Gibson

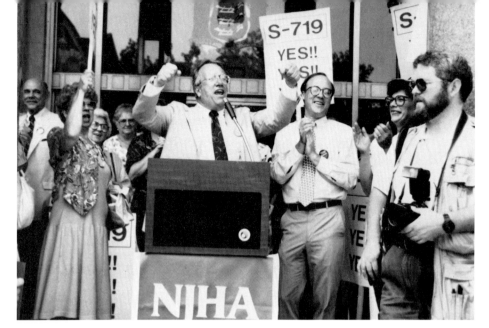

*N*JHA rallied to pass
S-719, an amendment to a
bill designed to protect the
pension and annuity
benefits of hospital
employees.
*Courtesy, New Jersey Hospital
Association*

*B*y their specialized
knowledge of medical
science, physicians gained
authority over lay
trustees, even in areas of
daily hospital routine.
*Courtesy, New Jersey Hospital
Association*

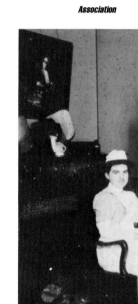

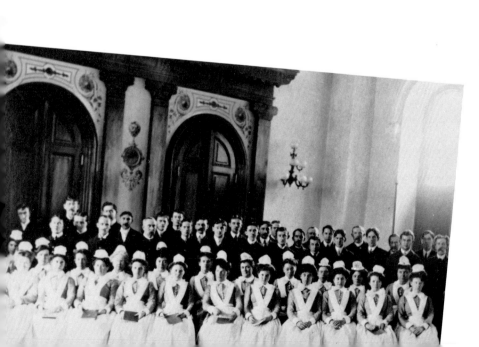

*A*s the complexity of
hospitals increased,
changes were needed in
such nonmedical areas as
building maintenance,
cleaning, and purchasing
supplies.
*Courtesy, New Jersey Hospital
Association*

*T*he need for specialized
education—given to these
training school students of
Greystone Psychiatric
Hospital in 1917—
continues to be a top
priority for hospitals.
*Courtesy, Greystone Park
Psychiatric Hospital*

and insubordination—as well as a black market in whiskey and tobacco, and activities such as card playing and gambling—flourished in the rambling households that were early hospitals.

Although physicians generally came from the same social class as the trustees and shared their view of a moral order, they had professional needs that sometimes clashed with the trustees' duty to protect society's dependents. Conflicts between physicians and trustees (and their surrogate, the superintendent) occurred over using patients in clinical teaching, performing autopsies, and admitting or discharging patients for medical rather than moral reasons. Even medical treatment might be a source of disagreement; trustees, as somber stewards, questioned the extravagant use of beef tea, new drugs, costly leeches "when a lancet would serve," and, especially, alcohol prescribed as a tonic or stimulant.

Throughout the 19th century, lay authorities maintained careful day-to-day control over every detail of hospital policies and procedures. Visiting committees, made up of members of the board of trustees, oversaw admissions, refusing patients who were incurable (these were referred to the Overseers of the Poor) or "unfit." Inspecting committees

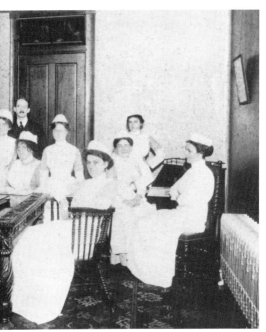

toured hospitals weekly to see that floors were scrubbed, walls white-washed, moldings dusted, blankets aired, and that "a proper economy" was observed. Any disobedience, profanity, or immorality—on the part of the patients or the house staff—was reported to the full board.

The Ascendancy of Physicians and Medical Science

By the time of the Civil War, however, the traditional view of hospital authority had begun to shift. The need for a full-time experienced physician to make emergency admissions and treat acute cases became increasingly apparent. By the mid-19th century, the office of resident physician had become accepted and even standardized. Inevitably, these administering physicians began to accumulate additional responsibilities, challenging the authority of the lay trustees in daily routines. Moreover, advances in medical education and medical treatment demanded an increasingly structured staff of physicians, quite different from the few part-time practitioners and partially trained students who intermittently visited the early hospitals and almshouses.

Because of the dramatic advances in medical science—especially in surgery—by the turn of the century, the

needs and perceptions of the medical profession began to dominate the hospitals. Hospitals became the physicians' "workshops"—almost their exclusive domains. The power and authority of the physicians increased further—and that of the trustees declined—as paying patients, brought in from the physicians' private practices, became a primary source of hospital revenue. Reflecting society's new reverence for science and efficiency, lay trustees had to adjust to the physicians' highly specialized knowledge and new professionalism. They began to play an increasingly passive and distant role, retreating from the hospitals' corridors and wards to the boardroom.

The Position and Power of the Hospital Administrator

Although medical responsibilities had been taken over by the medical staff, the overall operation of the hospital became increasingly complex. Recognizing the heavy responsibilities and highly specialized tasks required of hospital administrators, in 1899 a group formed the Association of Hospital Superintendents—the forerunner of the American Hospital Association—to exchange ideas concerning hospital management, economics, and operations. Soon thereafter, especially in the larger hospitals, the title "hospital superintendent," which implied only supervision, began to be replaced with "hospital administrator," which connoted initiative and leadership as well. The hospital standardization movement, launched in 1915 by the American College of Surgeons, affirmed the importance of the hospital administrator and the growing need for centralized control.

The demand for formal, specialized education and training at the university level became more and more apparent as well. The American College of Hospital Administrators (now the American College of Healthcare Executives), created in 1933, was especially instrumental in the development of university education for hospital administrators. The first degree-granting university program for hospital administration was begun in 1934 at the University of Chicago and continues to the present. Although the need for higher education for hospital administration had been recognized for years, the real demand came after World War II, when a number of programs were established in colleges and universities across the country.

The first empirical role study of the position of hospital administrator, conducted in 1945 with a grant from the Kellogg Foundation, resulted in a report intended to help establish a college curriculum in hospital administration. According to the report, hospital administration was more complicated than business administration because hospital executives often had conflicting allegiances—to the most advanced medical care, to the laws of economics, and to the needs of the community.

The role of the hospital administrator expanded in the 1960s with the implementation of the Great Society social legislation. Federal Medicare and Medicaid programs required hospitals to undertake a larger volume of service and document compliance with federal standards. A 1963 study of the administrator's role showed that departmental functioning—including nursing and special services—was the major concern of the hospital executive. By the mid-1960s, the hospital administrator—who now almost universally held the title of chief executive officer—had an established, agreed-upon role in the hospital, indisputably in charge of internal management. The 1970s saw more involvement of hospital CEOs in external affairs; they became more concerned with community relations, fund-raising, and interagency coordination, as well as attracting highly qualified physicians to the staff. Even with the strong hospital CEOs of the late 20th century, however, hospitals still show evidence of their three historic centers of authority. In the past, the relations among trustees, physicians, and administrators were seen from a monolithic view, in terms of power shifts. Now they are viewed in a more pluralistic way, in terms of power relationships.

New Roles and Accountabilities for Hospital Trustees

Today's healthcare system intensifies the need for the trustees' perspective and authority and gives new importance and meaning to their traditional functions: establishing long-term goals; planning facilities and services; providing for the financial resources to carry out the hospital's mission; and balancing the demands of patients, physicians, employees, government agencies, and third-party payors. While the trustees' authority has diminished in some areas, such as oversight of daily, internal procedures, it has expanded in others, such as representation of the hospital to external groups. Trustees have new roles, new responsibilities, and new legal accountabilities.

Traditionally, trustees have been the bridge between the hospital and the community, and this is true now more than ever. In the early days of America, the community shunned the hospital—usually placed outside of a town's geographical boundaries in remote areas—and its diseased and degraded inmates. Besides the house staff (who, like the patients, were usually society's outcasts) and the physicians, the only people who saw the inside of these institutions were the wealthy landowners, merchants, and town fathers who showed a beneficent interest. When the hospitals became the physicians' workshops, these centers of science and technology were inaccessible to laymen and trustees, and the community at large was alienated. Interestingly, the growth of insurance and prepayment plans in the second half of the 20th century caused a shift in the community's attitude toward the hospital. As people made payments in anticipation of someday needing hospital services, some of the mystery and awe began to fade and was replaced by a feeling of proprietorship. Also, with the increased involvement of hospital "outsiders"—government officials, insurance rate setters, lawyers, legislators, and community activists—came new areas of responsibility for trustees. Invariably, trustees, who previously stood at a distance as fiduciaries and fund-raisers, were drawn more into confrontation and negotiation—and legal liability.

Most of the new pressures on trustees came under the rubric of "accountability." In theory, trustees have always been accountable to the patients, families, and communities their hospitals serve. In reality, however, the duties of trustees were primarily to provide the facilities, equipment, and resources for physicians to treat the sick; they left responsibility for medical care to the medical professionals.

The actual role of trustees began to change in the 1960s when a series of court cases affirmed that hospitals—that is to say, their boards of trustees—have a duty that goes beyond delegating responsibility to the medical staff. In the landmark case of *Darling v. Charleston Community Memorial Hospital in* 1965, the Supreme Court of Illinois held the hospital corporation liable for not intervening through its administration to prevent the damage that occurred because of the negligence of the attending physician.

Recent decisions in Georgia, Nevada, Arizona, Montana, and Missouri have adopted a concept of the "corporate responsibility" of hospitals, implying legal liability for boards of trustees, either in whole or in part. The Supreme Court of Nevada, for example, ruled that "The hospital's role is no longer limited to the furnishing of physical facilities and equipment where a physician treats his private patients and practices his profession in his own individualized manner." Similarly, a court in Arizona ruled that a hospital's department of surgery had "acted for and on behalf of the hospital [in supervising the competence of its staff doctors], and if the department was negligent…then the hospital would also be negligent." Although the states that have affirmed the corporate responsibility of hospitals are still in a minority, many experts in the healthcare and legal fields predict that most major jurisdictions will adopt this concept in the future.

As they have been throughout their history, trustees are drawn from the most powerful and respected positions in society. Studies conducted by the American Hospital Association as well as several state hospital associations show that one-half to two-thirds of all hospital trustees are bankers, lawyers, corporate executives, and entrepreneurs. Since governing bodies in the 1990s, however, are "working boards" and not honorary enclaves, trustees in these fields are valued for their economic and business knowledge more than for their influence and prestige. Professionals in such fields as public relations, marketing, and communications are also sought for their specialized expertise. "Community representatives" have increased, although perhaps more slowly than expected. More women—especially professional women—serve on boards. The major change that has occurred in the composition of boards is the greater number of physicians that serve as trustees, since traditional barriers to their membership have been lowered. Also, the hospital's chief executive officer is increasingly a voting board member, usually with the title of "president," rather than serving as the board's servant or delegate.

Boards have become smaller than in the past. Although it varies greatly depending on the type of hospital, the average board has 15 trustees. Boards and their committees meet more often and for longer periods of time; trustees spend about 10 to 15 hours a month in meetings. About 90 percent of hospital trustees—unlike their counterparts in business and industry—receive no compensation for their service, although 60 percent are reimbursed for expenses. Moreover, while at one time it was not unusual for appointments to be for life, trustees in the 1990s tend to have fixed terms. Attendance—and, more crucially, performance—are required of modern hospital trustees.

In New Jersey, urban, suburban, and rural hospitals across the state illustrate the changing trends in modern hospital governance and management. Elizabeth General Medical Center, an urban hospital in the industrialized northern part of the state, has a board of trustees consisting of 25 members, drawn from leaders in the community. This is a diverse group, with trustees representing different areas of expertise and interest from airports to banking to pharmaceuticals. Trustees are active in every aspect of the hospital; three-quarters of the trustees serve on board committees, including credentialing, capital budget, planning, and quality of care. Public affairs is an especially important area of board activity; trustees speak, testify, and write letters to legislators on important hospital issues. As an urban hospital that serves a large population of uninsured and medically indigent people, Elizabeth General Medical Center sees the issue of uncompensated care as an especially pressing concern facing New Jersey as well as the nation.

At the other end of the state, The Memorial Hospital of Salem County, a 150-bed rural hospital located in the sparsely populated southern area, has a board of 20 trustees representing a cross-section of the community. One of the most important board committees oversees physician credentialing. While the Memorial Hospital of Salem County is a small, rural hospital, it must remain competitive with metropolitan hospitals in Philadelphia and Wilmington, just across New Jersey's borders.

In 1951, employees posed in front of newly opened Valley Hospital in Ridgewood. The hospital admitted 3,704 patients its first year and now admits over 30,000.
Courtesy, The Valley Hospital

Morristown Memorial Hospital, a suburban hospital in northern New Jersey, has three boards of trustees: a foundation, or parent, board of 15 members; an 11-member board for the hospital's affiliated for-profit corporation; and a hospital board consisting of 25 members. Trustees for the boards are selected to represent a variety of professions and occupations as well as a diverse geographical area. The hospital has a membership corporation of 135 people representing an even broader cross-section of the community. While this body can be compared to the stockholders, or shareholders, of a corporation, in another way the institution's organization is traditionally that of a hospital—the medical staff is a distinct entity, reporting directly to the board of trustees.

Another suburban hospital, Somerset Medical Center, has a large board of 55 trustees, 10 of whom serve as ex officio members, to ensure that all areas and interests of the community are represented. Somerset, like most hospitals of today, stresses the need for its trustees to have an understanding of healthcare in general, as well as an awareness of the high expectations that modern consumers have of hospitals—especially in the northeastern region of the country. The Valley Hospital, a suburban hospital in Ridgewood, has a relatively small board of a maximum of 25 members, selected to bring special skills in areas such as management, law, finance, investments, and insurance; volunteers and physicians also serve. Typical of members of a "working board," trustees also serve on committees, including ethics, quality control, technology assessment, and fund-raising. The board directly oversees The Valley Hospital's auxiliary, a separate fund-raising branch of 2,500 volunteers.

As the role of the trustee has evolved into such a demanding and time-consuming position of responsibility, trustee development programs are required by JCAHO and are almost universally offered by hospitals. Although the depth and content of activities vary greatly among institutions, a comprehensive board development program consists of a continuing process of education, often beginning before the trustee is officially appointed, and continuing through

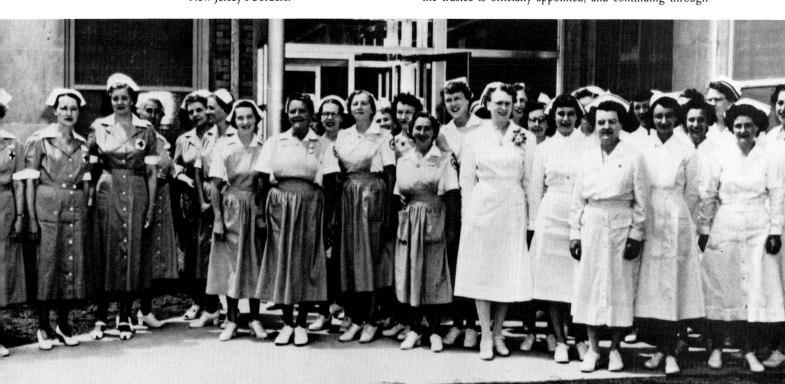

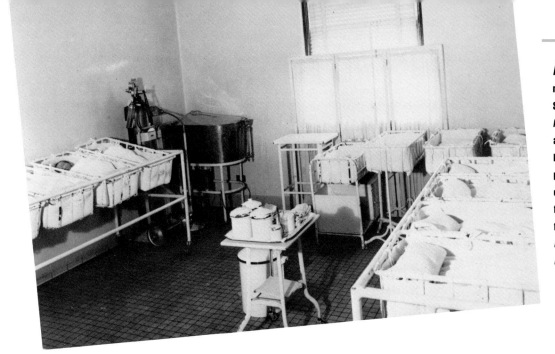

*B*ehind the serenity of the maternity ward of Somerset Hospital, opened August 1925, administrators had to balance the needs of patients, physicians, and employees with the financial resources to pay for them.

Courtesy, Somerset Medical Center

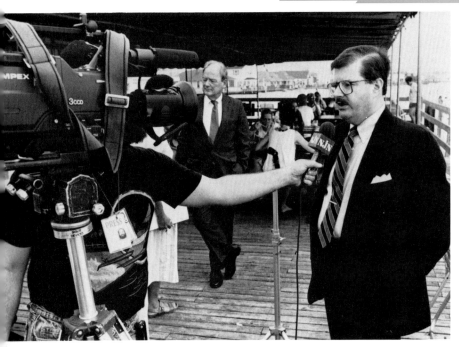

*A*n NJHA official addresses the press in a "clean beach" campaign to educate the public that New Jersey hospitals follow stringent requirements for waste disposal.

Courtesy, New Jersey Hospital Association

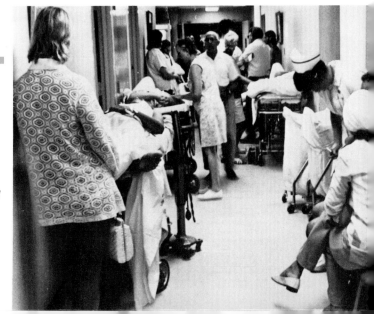

*A*lready complex hospital payment systems became even more complicated with the introduction of federal Medicare and Medicaid programs.

Courtesy, New Jersey Hospital Association

tenure on the board. Robert Wood Johnson University Hospital, a large teaching hospital, provides an excellent example of a state-of-the-art program of board training and development, as well as board self-examination and preparation.

A goal of both the American Hospital Association and the New Jersey Hospital Association has been to increase the active participation of trustees in the state association. Such involvement in the work of NJHA, through the Council on Hospital Governance, helps meet the informational need of individual board members from hospitals across the state, while allowing the association to benefit from the expertise and perspective of the trustees. Each year, three members of NJHA's board are hospital trustees, and may also serve on board committees, councils, advisory groups, and task forces. Educational programs and materials for hospital trustees are developed through the NJHA's Health Research and Educational Trust.

Today's Hospitals—"Businesslike" but Not Businesses

The new accountabilities of trustees as well as a host of other trends—including the increasing power of hospital CEOs, the development of multiunit hospitals, and the demands of competition and the marketplace—raises the question of the identity of hospitals: Are they, or should they be, operated as "businesses" in a healthcare "industry"? Historically, differences of mission (to render service rather than accumulate money) and structure (separate, distinct centers of authority rather than a clear hierarchy) obscured the many similarities between hospitals and businesses. In fact, because of their emphasis on charity, good management practices in hospitals were often considered irrelevant or even suspect. Before World War II, cost accounting was unknown and was even viewed as unseemly in most hospitals. In keeping with the perception of hospitals as a charitable enterprise quite different from business, the staff, especially nurses, residents, and orderlies, were generally underpaid and overworked.

In recent decades, hospitals—much to their benefit and perhaps even for their survival—have borrowed management concepts and learned from business and industry. Yet hospitals have never succeeded in governing their institutions like corporations, factories, or department stores, and in New Jersey there is a growing consensus that this would not be desirable even if it were feasible. A hospital's transactions involve health and sickness, life and death, pain and caring; its "products" are beyond accounting. The operation of hospitals is far more complicated than that of other enterprises; students of management have described the task of running hospitals as the most complex in society. While the management of hospitals must include sound principles of business and management, it must also go beyond them.

NJHA has taken a leadership role in New Jersey, setting an example for the country, in initiating discussion on hospital management and business practices. A Joint Task Force on Hospital Business Ethics, formed by NJHA's Councils on Governance and Management Practices, hosted an invitational symposium of experts in the spring of 1992. As a result of this groundbreaking endeavor, NJHA prepared a statement of principles for New Jersey hospitals to use as a model for adopting their own guidelines for business practices. Precisely because hospitals are not like for-profit enterprises, special attention must be paid to the ethical framework of business ventures and relationships. Routine business practices such as diversification, customer satisfaction, financial leveraging, venture start-up capitalization, business loans, and competitive executive compensation take on new meaning in the context of hospitals. The underlying issue is not what hospitals do, but what hospitals are. By the very nature of their unique history and mission, hospitals are ethical enterprises.

Healthcare professionals in New Jersey, under the leadership of NJHA, have come to a consensus that hospitals must establish careful, effective, and fair business practices, looking after their resources carefully to ensure that they are well spent. At the same time, hospitals must transcend business considerations. Because of the intimate and critical way in which they touch people's lives at times of great vulnerability—and because of the circumstances of their founding and operation—hospitals have forged a covenant or compact with their communities. The public has a special expectation of fairness and trustworthiness, and needs to have faith in hospitals' business practices, in order to have confidence in their clinical practices as well. NJHA's *Guidelines for Adoption of a Statement of Hospital Business Ethics* represents a codification of ethical business issues as currently understood and—perhaps more importantly—provides a basis for continuing dialogue.

State Legislation and Regulation

Hospitals are major forces of the communities they serve. As complex organizations with complex roles, a wide range of laws affect the operations of hospitals, including those covering nonprofit corporations; civil and criminal justice; statutes of limitations; labor and workers' compensation; claims for payment; maintenance of and access to medical records; birth and death certificates; safe handling of food, drugs, and narcotics; public health; operation of passenger elevators, steam generators, and boilers; and even the conduct of fund-raising bingo games and raffles.

Yet even more regulations cover professional licensing and the practice of medicine and the duties, obligations, and activities of physicians, nurses, dietitians, midwives, pharmacists, occupational therapists, physical therapists, social workers, respiratory care workers, and other healthcare professionals who make a hospital work. Regulations also govern the means by which healthcare organizations receive approval to build new facilities, offer new services, and finance improvements.

As the level and cost of care has risen, regulation of healthcare has steadily increased. Regulations tend to be imposed as solutions to problems—of quality, accessibility or costs, for example. At different times in history, more regulation has been instituted to ensure the safety, health, and well-being of citizens and healthcare workers whose knowledge and dedication keep hospitals running. Other legislative efforts have been sought to increase hospital efficiency, enhance quality of care, and contain healthcare costs.

New Jersey has used the political process and passed legislation that established buildings, programs, and principles of progressive and humane healthcare. Today, at any point in time, scores of bills are before the state legislature addressing healthcare needs and affecting the hospital industry in New Jersey. Keeping up-to-date on those bills and representing the interests of hospitals to the legislature, is just one of the many roles of the New Jersey Hospital Association.

Members of NJHA's numerous councils—on auxiliaries, finance, hospital governance, management practices, planning, professional practice, education, and government relations—are healthcare professionals who work in hospitals. The councils are active participants in the association's decision-making process. After studying proposed legislation, the appropriate council makes recommendations to the association's board of directors and to the Council on Government Relations, which represents the association's official position on a proposed bill. When appropriate, committees and task forces are formed to study particularly difficult issues and to reach a consensus opinion that is acceptable to a broad base of hospitals statewide.

Reforming Healthcare

New Jersey, along with the rest of the nation, continues its struggle to formulate healthcare policies that meet the varied needs of a diverse public—the consumer, provider, insurer, employer, and hospital. In the numerous approaches to healthcare reform, some call for less regulation and some for more.

In mid-1989, NJHA President Louis P. Scibetta created the President's Task Force on Regulatory Reform, one of the most significant interdisciplinary efforts of NJHA in the last decade. The Executive Committee of the NJHA Board of Trustees and 17 hospital chief executives and trustees from throughout the state formed the President's Task Force and were charged with developing an overview of the healthcare regulatory scene and presenting a blueprint for improvement.

The result of their analysis was published in July 1990 and presented to Governor Jim Florio's Commission of Health Care Costs. Aptly entitled, "Hospital Regulation at the Turning Point: Opportunities for Change," the document suggests that government has become too involved in the management of hospitals.

"Instead of managing rate setting, government often winds up micro-managing hospitals," the report states. "This must change. Intimate involvement, through excessive regulation, in the day-to-

day management activities of hospitals is not government's role. Such a process is time consuming, costly and counterproductive. On the federal level alone it is estimated that $50 billion of the $600 billion spent on healthcare yearly is associated with regulatory 'administrative costs.' On the state level, if the same ratio is applied, the cost would be an added $50 million annually, and this is no doubt a conservative estimate."

NJHA, through the report, made 28 specific recommendations on policy development, the overall financial environment of the hospital industry in New Jersey, uncompensated care, access to care and insurance, a new rate-setting structure and process, issues of planning, alternate care services and facilities, and tort reform to reduce frivolous and costly law suits and therefore the cost of malpractice insurance.

The NJHA President's Task Force recommended that the hospital regulatory system embrace certain goals, among them that "citizens get the hospital care that's needed; hospitals provide that care efficiently at the most reasonable cost to the consumer; hospitals' operating and capital needs are met; outpatient and alternative care settings are promoted; regulators must be anticipatory, developing a 'big picture' plan for the state, directed by policy; and the needs of the uninsured and underinsured are met."

Yet another approach to healthcare reform is embodied in the State Health Plan unveiled in late 1991 by the State Health Planning Board of the New Jersey Department of Health. The plan, initially approved by state regulators in March, was met with public protest, centered around the proposed closing of numerous hospitals and hospital units.

While the state has been involved in health planning for some time, the State Health Plan has taken on increased importance since the 1991 Health Care Cost Reduction Act, which shifted the nature of the document from one of a planning paper to one bearing the weight of regulation.

Among the suggestions of the plan, which was published as a regulatory document but now has been down-

NJHA President Louis P. Scibetta (at front) and George F. Lynn, president of Atlantic City Medical Center, educate legislators about issues pertinent to NJHA and hospitals across the country.
Courtesy, New Jersey Hospital Association

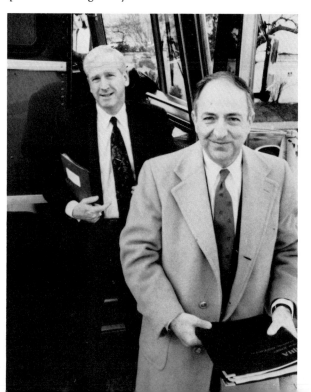

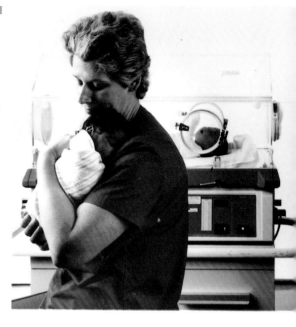

Highly specialized intensive care provides extra attention for newborns at Somerset Medical Center's Maternity Care Center.
Courtesy, Somerset Medical Center

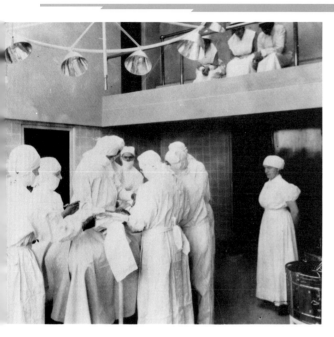

Like no other industry, the purpose of healthcare services has remained the same from the beginning— to offer care in the most effective manner using the best medical technology available.
Courtesy, Barnert Hospital

Speaking at the annual meeting, New Jersey Governor Jim Florio listened to NJHA recommendations that helped shape the Health Care Reform Act, designed to assure access to care for all.
Courtesy, New Jersey Hospital Association

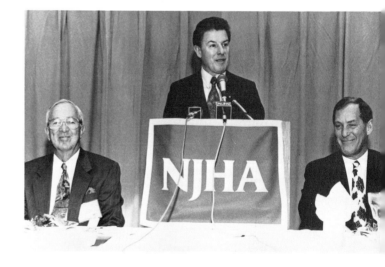

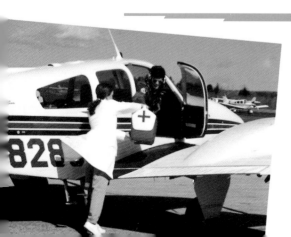

As medical science perfects organ and tissue transplants, the procedures become even more controversial because of the expense, low availability, and coordination of allocation.
Photo by L. O'Shaughnessy/ Medichrome

graded to one that is "advisory" only, the Department of Health called for the closing of 25 pediatric units, six hospitals, and the reduction, consolidation, or elimination of obstetrical beds in 16 hospitals.

The proposed cuts in hospital services and capacity were requested as cost-containment measures. If the negative response of the public and the healthcare community is any indication, yardsticks other than cost need to be applied before closing or limiting services. NJHA and its hospital members continue to advocate a health planning process that begins with local input and works its way up the state hierarchy to the Department of Health, rather than going downward as decrees from the state.

Hospital Governance and Leadership in a Changing World

No other institution in America has undergone such complete transformation as hospitals. Moreover, healthcare in New Jersey and in the nation is facing more rapid change, escalating complexity, and difficult choices than ever before. A few predictions that will affect the governance of tomorrow's hospitals are:

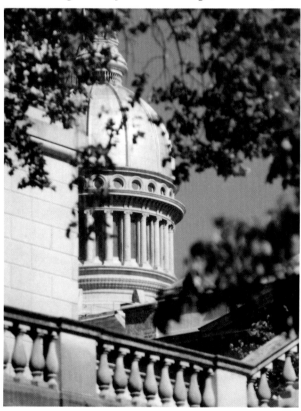

- Hospitals will increasingly be controlled by outside forces.
- Healthcare delivery will be more sophisticated and expensive.
- Some type of nationalized health insurance will be initiated.
- There will be fewer small hospitals, but more multiunit facilities and sharing of resources.
- Outpatient services will become increasingly popular.

- Hospitals will become centers of "wellness," or preventive care—the next great frontier in healthcare.

As hospitals prepare for the next century, New Jersey, with leadership from NJHA, will continue to demonstrate the state's characteristic inventiveness and innovation. New Jersey will initiate model programs and new ideas, and it will provide a leading example of the process by which the future can be confidently faced. Since its founding 75 years ago, NJHA has been committed to providing a forum for healthcare issues. In 1918, seven hospital executives first came together to discuss common concerns facing New Jersey's hospitals. Today there are many more "players" and the issues are far more complex. Not only hospital executives, trustees, and physicians, but government officials, legislators, business leaders, labor representatives, scholars, educators, communicators, and citizens of the community are concerned with healthcare. Major issues they will discuss—at the forum provided by NJHA—will include the cost and financing of healthcare, ensuring quality and access of care for all, providing care for the needy and uninsured, resolving the inequities in the hospital billing system, and revising the Medicare payment policy. Participants will bring their own agendas, perceptions, and priorities, all of which are vital to building the future of hospitals and healthcare. The time has come in New Jersey and in the nation, says Louis P. Scibetta, president of NJHA, to work together and to write new chapters of history. "There must be participation of everyone involved. And healthcare involves *everyone*."

*H*ealthcare leaders across the country watch activities at the New Jersey State Capitol in Trenton.
Photo by Mark E. Gibson

*P*hysicians and hospital administrators constantly work with changing legislation—so healthcare professionals like this physical therapist can most effectively do their jobs.
Photo by Mark E. Gibson

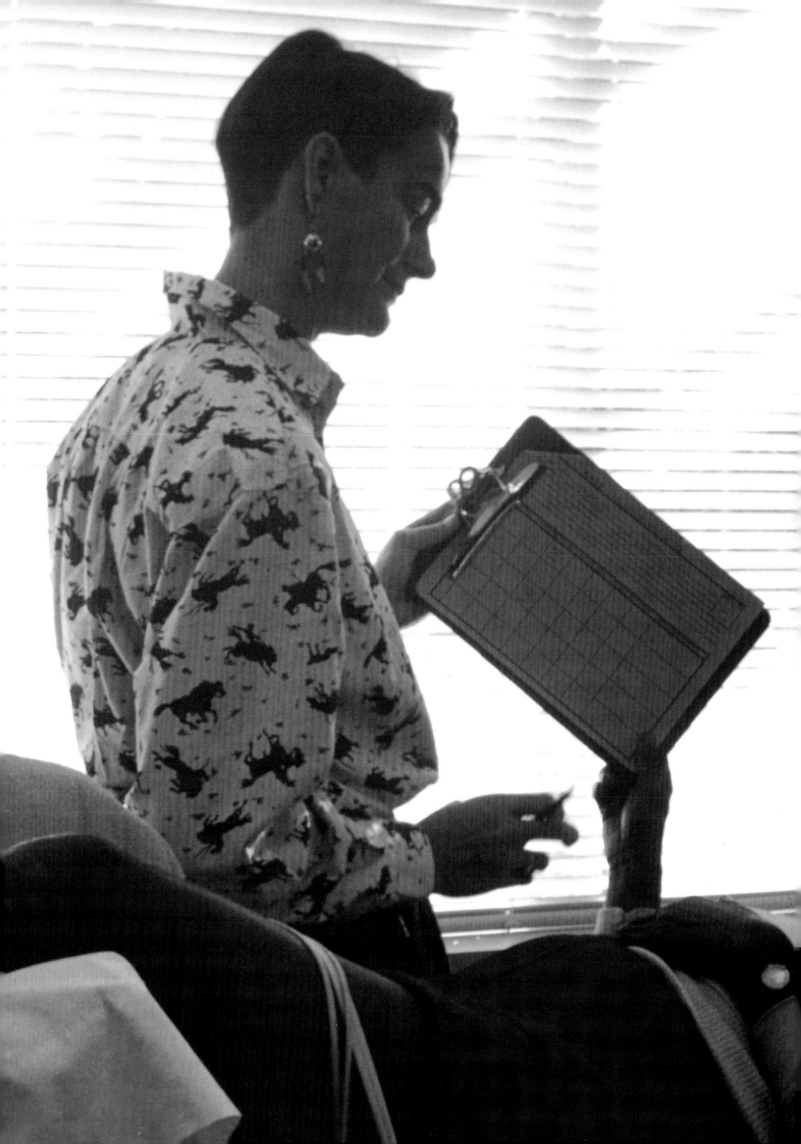

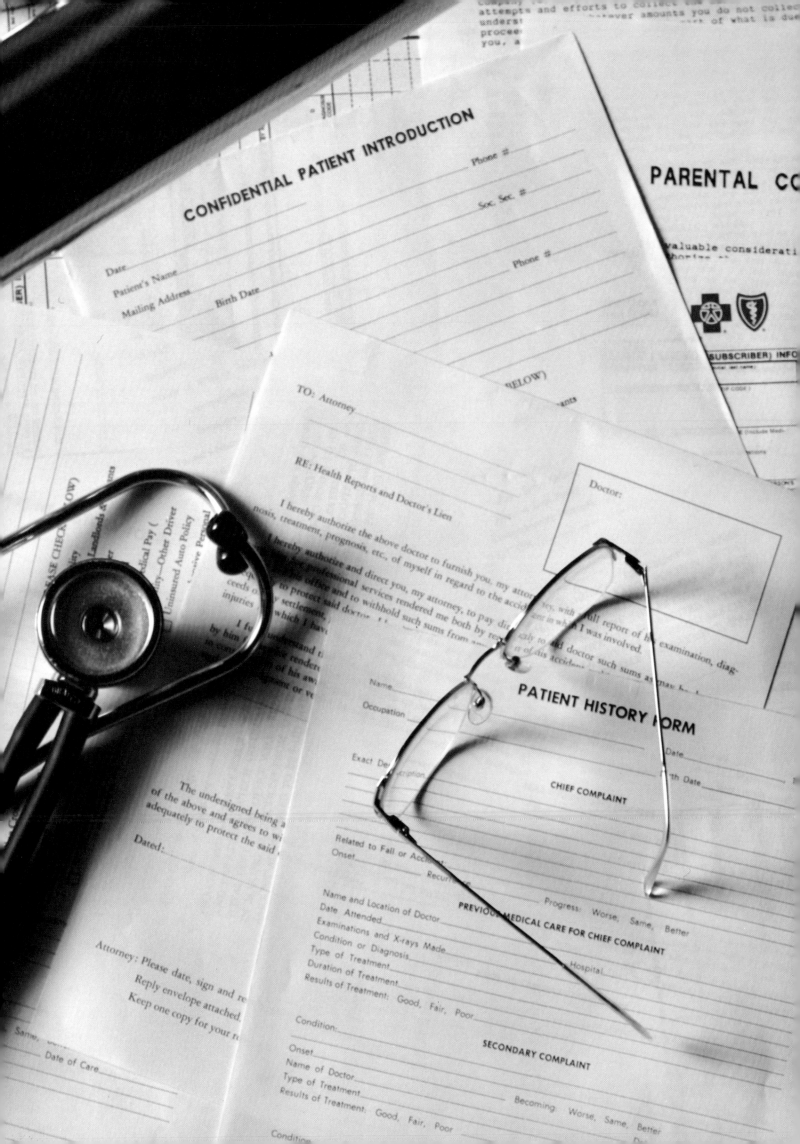

The issue of how to pay hospitals for the services they provide has challenged New Jersey to create systems that fairly meet the different needs of patient, hospital, and payor—namely, insurance plans. Over the years, numerous solutions have been developed, tested, and discarded. New Jersey is once again at a critical point in history. In a federal court, Judge Alfred M. Wolin ruled that certain elements of the New Jersey reimbursement system in place since 1978 are preempted by the federal Employee Retirement and Income Security Act (ERISA). The shifting of costs of those who cannot pay to those who can is illegal for members of self-funded health plans.

According to a nationally recognized hospital rate lawyer, "Whether it gets reversed or doesn't get reversed, the Wolin decision has crystalized a number of issues and forced them to the front. Society says everyone should have access to high-quality healthcare; but we have not come to grips with how we pay for those individuals who do not have access. Employers and self-funded insurance plans are looking for a way to reduce the amount of healthcare cost shifts they are willing to bear. They are saying they can no longer afford this."

Late in 1992, a new system replaced the current payment system based on Diagnostic Related Groups (DRGs). Once again, New Jersey had the opportunity to blend expertise and innovation to create a means to reimburse hospitals—a solution that works for all and allows the hospitals to remain economically viable while continuing to provide citizens with high quality medical care.

H O S P I T A L
P A Y M E N T
S Y S T E M S

Equitable Solutions toward Healthcare for All

Early Cost-Control Efforts

Since hospitals at the turn of the century were charity institutions, often affiliated with religious organizations, they provided free care to the sick and needy. The more well-to-do citizens were nursed and cared for at home, often by family members. As medicine advanced and hospitals could offer more services, paying patients were admitted.

In the nascent years of NJHA, hospitals were already grappling with economic issues of being compensated for the care they provided. Throughout the 1930s and 1940s, care for the indigent was a large concern of hospitals and, therefore, NJHA. At a 1936 meeting of NJHA, a professor from New York University addressed the group on the role of the hospital in community life and cautioned that "hospitals fail to meet the needs of the entire populace, in that they have not solved the problem of caring for the indigent without branding them as paupers, and of providing suitable care at a reasonable cost for middle-class patients."

A 1941 NJHA president's address by F. Stanley Howe, is typical of the concerns of that era: "Until the unquestioned right of the hospital to be protected in its losses on the care of indigent citizens has been definitely established, we shall continue to lead a precarious existence, especially with the rising costs, both of commodities and services."

Hospitals considered it the duty of municipalities to contribute sufficient money to hospitals for the full care of those unable to pay, however, hospitals believed that private patients should not pay more than their share to meet the deficit of "ward cases."

One of the first attempts to control hospital costs and provide hospitals with adequate payment was instituted in 1938 when the New Jersey legislature established the Hospital Health Service Plan of New Jersey, or Blue Cross, as it came to be known, a cooperative effort of 17 hospitals. Operated in the public interest, Blue Cross was exempt from state and federal taxes, and, for all practical purposes, was a public company.

As a new kind of noncommercial, not-for-profit insurer, Blue Cross was to provide full payment directly to participating hospitals for services that its subscribers received. Blue Cross rates were the same to all subscribers, regardless of their risk, making hospitalization insurance more affordable to a wider public. Blue Cross and hospitals had a symbiotic relationship. Blue Cross depended on hospitals' acceptance of it, and hospitals counted many Blue Cross subscribers among their patients.

But Blue Cross also had a special relationship with the state for many years as the only regulated payor. At the same time Blue Cross was established, the Commissioner of Banking and Insurance was charged with regulating hospital rates that were fair to both hospitals and Blue Cross subscribers. Throughout the 1940s and into the 1950s, the hospital rate-setting process for Blue Cross was rather informal. Hospitals asked the commissioner for approval of rates above predetermined ceilings, and almost routinely received waivers.

According to *Historical Perspective of Hospital Rate-Setting in New Jersey*, a 1976 NJHA publication, "The hospital interest in a responsible approach to spending limits had its New Jersey origins in 1956—a year in which such thoughts would have been regarded as heretical almost anywhere else. At that time, institutions agreed

to work with then Commissioner of Banking and Insurance Charles R. Howell to contain the expense. Howell feared that if rates exceeded $28 [per day], it would have the effect of pricing hospital service out of the market."

A peer review process helped keep costs in check and involved hospital trustees, administrators, physicians, and government officials as well as health consumers.

Reimbursement and Restrictions

Medicaid, providing healthcare for the nation's poor, and Medicare, ensuring healthcare for the elderly, became law in the 1960s, and marked the beginning of a new era of hospital regulation, which was made more complex by the introduction of yet another regulatory influence—the federal government.

As Jack W. Owen, then executive vice president and director of NJHA, wrote in the association's 1966-67 annual report: "The big event, of course, was the implementation of Public Law 89-97, more commonly referred to as Medicare....I need not elaborate the problems of Medicare since most of you are familiar with the clerical billing and medical specialist problems. All of this activity required many meetings, negotiations, and communications. Not all of our problems are solved, nor do we anticipate that next year will answer all the questions."

Proposed by NJHA, an 11-member committee to advise the commissioner began to review hospital budgets in 1968 for the fiscal year approaching. The committee made cost-saving suggestions, and approved hardship cases for hospitals to receive payment above fixed ceiling rates. Hospital trustees, administrators, and physicians participated in a peer review process designed to help contain costs.

The next year, the work of the advisory committee fell to the Health Research and Educational Trust (HRET) of New Jersey under the umbrella of the Hospital Budget and Cost Review Program, serving the New Jersey Department of Insurance in its responsibility to review and approve hospital budgets for reimbursement purposes. HRET had been founded in 1964 as a nonprofit corporate affiliate of NJHA to engage in research and education activities focused on issues in healthcare delivery, use, costs, and operations.

In May and December of 1969, however, two requests for rate increases by Blue Cross, which would have raised its premiums 73 percent, prompted an examination of hospital rate setting. The result of this examination was published in the *Wharton Report*, named for the head of the study commission, T. Girard Wharton.

Wharton criticized the lack of consumer representation on the advisory committee, the

ST. PETER'S GENERAL HOSPITAL
From November 8, 1907, to December 31, 1908

The following Report is respectfully submitted by the Sisters of St Peter's Hospital.

	Male	Female	Total
Number of patients admitted	194	192	386
Number of patients discharged cured	168	169	337
Number of patients discharged improved	6	3	9
Number of patients unimproved		3	3
Number of deaths	12	6	18
Number of patients remaining in the institution December 31, 1908	8	11	19
	194	192	386

Average days' stay of patients, 19 days per patient.

Collective days' stay of patients in the institution, 7457.

Average cost per day per patient, $1.40.

Number of pay patients, 186.

Number of free patients, 200.

review process of rate making, and the retrospective quality of cost reviews. "The review has always taken place after the expenses have been incurred, making it very difficult for the advisory committee to disallow items, as it realized the money had already been spent," according to the report.

Many hospital cost controls proposed by the *Wharton Report* are in use today, including preadmission testing, competitive bidding for services, and joint purchasing policies for hospitals. The report also explored the per-case method of hospital reimbursement and contrasted it with the per-diem method, which is based on the daily rate hospitals traditionally charged to cover most institutional expenses of hospitalization, including food, linens, nursing, routine lab, X-ray, and medical supplies.

Numerous measures attempted to establish adequate and consistent rate reimbursements for hospitals. And while rate increases for Blue Cross, the primary insurer in the state, were denied, other insurers, a smaller group of companies representing fewer patients, were forced to bear the costs that Blue Cross couldn't pay. Cost-shifting occurred and inequities of payment grew.

In a *Health Affairs* article (Spring 1984) that outlines the New Jersey DRG system, James A. Morone and Andrew Dunham wrote: "When hospital inflation began to quicken in the early 1960s, the commissioner [of insurance] discovered that approving higher premiums meant media criticism. Blue Cross officials began to argue that the political pressures limiting their premiums should be offset by similar limits to what they paid to hospitals."

The Sweeping Changes of the 1970s

Since early attempts to control hospital costs did not succeed, in 1971, the state legislature passed the Health Care Facilities Planning Act, giving the State Departments of Health and Insurance unprecedented power over the health-care industry in New Jersey. Along with the Commissioners of Health and Insurance, a new Health Care Administration Board (HCAB) was established to see that the act was implemented.

The Commissioner of Health was charged with approving hospital charges to the state Medicaid program and, along with the Commissioner of Insurance, was responsible for regulating charges to Blue Cross. In addition, the Department of Health was to assure that all healthcare facilities used a uniform accounting system, in a sense giving it authority to scrutinize line items of hospitals' budgets and make judgments about the efficiency of healthcare delivery.

Then in 1974, a Princeton-based public-interest research group —the Center for the Analysis of Public Issues—published a report, "Bureaucratic Malpractice," which criti-

***M**any blame the use of high technology— not as prevalent in 1941—for rising costs. But operating expenses, salaries, administration, facilities, and consumer demand all add to medical care inflation.*
Courtesy, Zurbrugg Hospital/Graduate Health System, Inc.

Mr. Charles Gerken

Debtor to ZURBRUGG MEMORIAL HOSPITA

To rent of room	$ 4.50
To use of operating room	6.00
To use of delivery room	
To baby's board	
To special nurse's board	
To laboratory	5.00
To telephone	
To X-ray	
To special prescription	
To extras	
	$15.50

RECEIVED PAYMENT
ZURBRUGG MEMORIAL HOSP.

All bills payable at office weekly in advance

***N**JHA helps disseminate information through publications (left) and the Health Research and Educational Trust Corporate Information Center (right).*
Courtesy, New Jersey Hospital Association

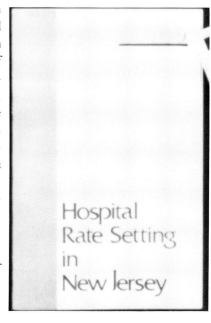

Hospital
Rate Setting
in
New Jersey

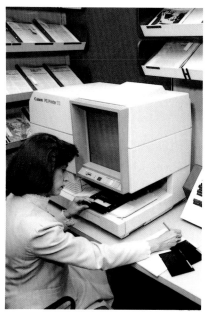

cized the state for permitting an industry to regulate itself. The newly installed administration of Governor Brendan T. Byrne immediately seized upon the momentum of the report and took control of the hospital rate review system.

"Though it had the statutory authority to do so, it [the state] had not yet developed the competence," according to Morone and Dunham in *Health Affairs*. "State officials even had to borrow forms from the hospital association. Confusion, conflict, and long delays—the most painful concomitants of hastily imposed regulation—marked the system for several years as the state scrambled to define and implement its rate review methodology."

In 1974, the HRET advisory committee that reviewed hospital budgets and costs was terminated. The Department of Health was required by law to perform this function. During its four years of operation, the committee had reviewed more than 150 hospital budgets and in the process saved more than $70.3 million in healthcare costs.

The years of 1974, '75 and '76 were fraught with uncertainty and confusion. A 1976 publication of HRET, *Son of Gobbledegook…Hospital Rate-Setting in New Jersey* (making reference to a Maryland judge's opinion of that state's hospital rate-approval guidelines, which were based on formulas similar to New Jersey's), describes the rate-setting process: "The rates are inadequate….The formula ignores law, regulations, contracts, and a host of other realities hospitals must function within."

Further citing an example of nurse-patient staffing ratios: "In recent months, a number of New Jersey hospitals were inspected in this regard, and subsequently told to increase the number of nurses employed in order to meet the state's licensure requirements. These same hospitals, however, had also been told by the department's rate-setting staff, that they would have to decrease the number of nurses employed."

When computers at the Department of Health produced a rate increase of only 2 1/2 percent over 1974 for 1975, NJHA and hospitals protested and in the end, the state conceded that "reasonable" rates were more appropriate at a 13 percent increase. Other court cases by NJHA and individual institutions resulted in settlements and some financial relief for hospitals.

It took until the mid-1970s for the state to institute standard financial reporting for hospitals. New Jersey's complex per-diem rate-setting program was known as SHARE (Standard Hospital Accounting and Rate Evaluation). But SHARE applied only to Blue Cross and Medicaid payments, at that time the limit of the state's jurisdiction.

"Blue Cross and Medicaid payments were tightly controlled. However, hospitals protected their cash flow by simply shifting costs to the unregulated payors, particularly the commercial insurers….The differential between Blue Cross payments to hospitals and those of other payors reached 30 percent within five years….The burden of uncompensated care also had to be shifted to commercial and private payors," wrote Morone and Dunham.

The economic problems of hospitals continued to intensify. Then NJHA President Jack Owen, in the association's 1976 annual report wrote: "The rate-setting dilemma continues to worsen. Not only were rates set by the Department of Health woefully inadequate…but the appeals processes were reduced to a charade….One of the major elements of our frustration was, and continues to be, the inflexibility of our formula by which the so-called 'economic factor' is determined and applied to rate increases."

The SHARE program was criticized for not recognizing the difference between hospitals and for not reimbursing hospitals adequately. According to NJHA's 1977 annual report, "Corrections to the SHARE system resulted in approximately $29 million in adjustments to the 1977 payment rates."

Additionally, the per-diem rate structure gave hospitals little incentive to provide quality care efficiently. Perhaps recognizing that, the New Jersey Department of Health was experimenting with the concept of Diagnostic Related Groups, using a reimbursement per-case rate as a basis for setting hospital industry rates.

By 1978, some temporary relief in rates was found in revision of SHARE guidelines. That year's NJHA annual report describes: "As a result of two years of discussion and review involving the Department of Health, Blue Cross, Commercial Insurance Carriers and economists employed on behalf of the industry, [NJHA] was able to persuade the department to increase their original economic factor by developing a more accurate and equitable method of identifying inflation."

S-446 —Yet Another New Way to Reimburse Hospitals

Escalating hospital costs were not just a problem in New Jersey but nationwide, as many states searched for a reimbursement method that would compensate hospitals fairly while moderating the growth of expenditures.

On July 20, 1978, a law enacted by the State of New Jersey, S-446, substantially changed the Health Care Facilities Planning Act of 1971. New Jersey instituted yet another system for reimbursing hospitals—an all-payor, prospective system.

Previously, the Commissioner of Health was authorized to set rates for Blue Cross and Medicaid patients, limiting hospital costs for some 42 percent of those using hospital services. Now the state's rate-setting power was extended to control hospital rates for privately insured persons and the

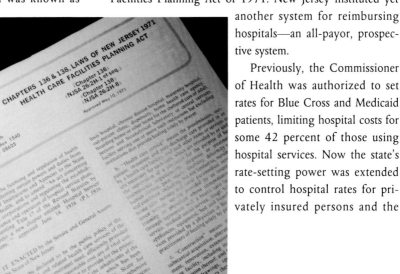

The morass of claim forms and billing procedures—along wi uncertainties about insurance coverage—leading consumers and healthcare profession: toward major reform. Photo by John Riley/Medichrome

The 1971 Health Car Facilities Planning Act authorized the New Je Department of Health impose a uniform accounting system on hospitals in the state. Courtesy, the New Jerse Department of Health

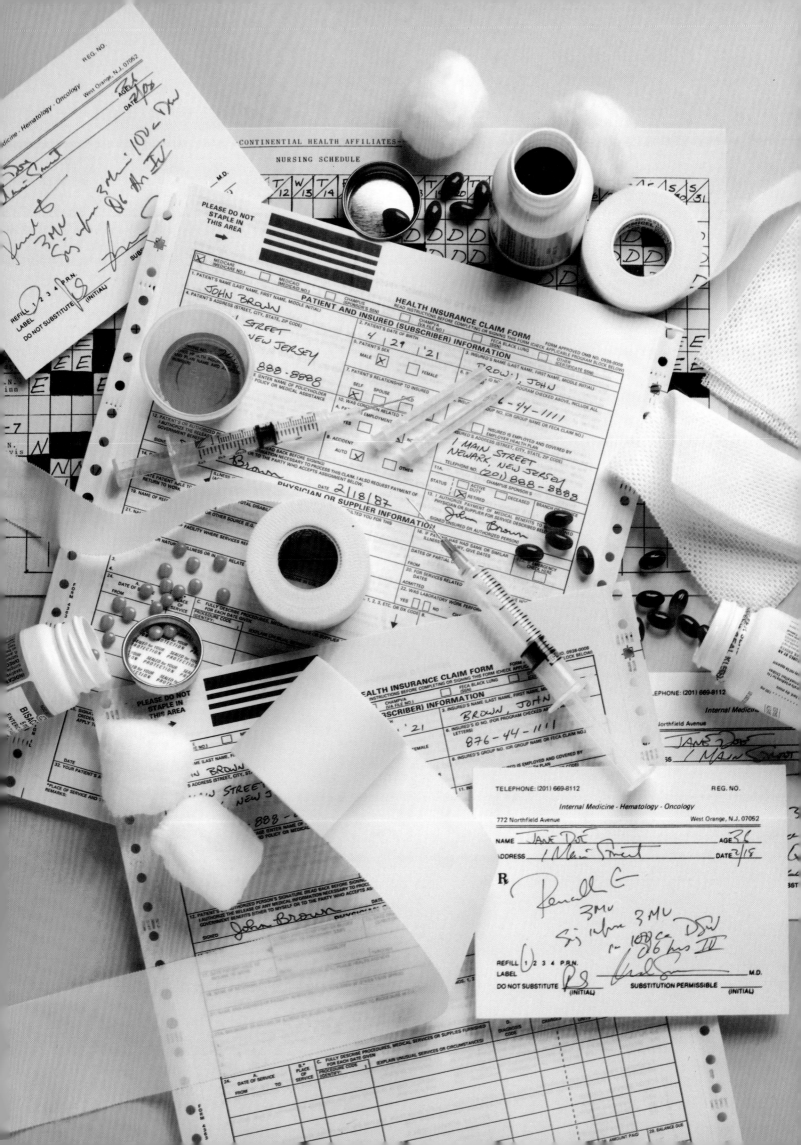

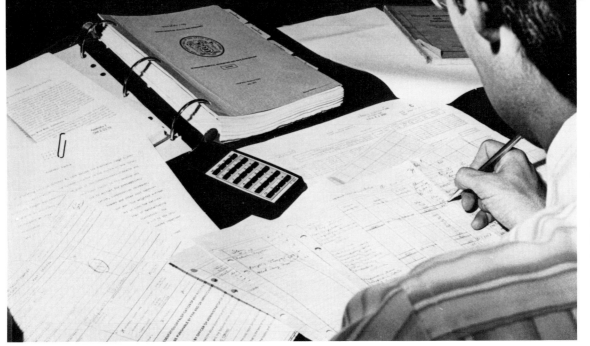

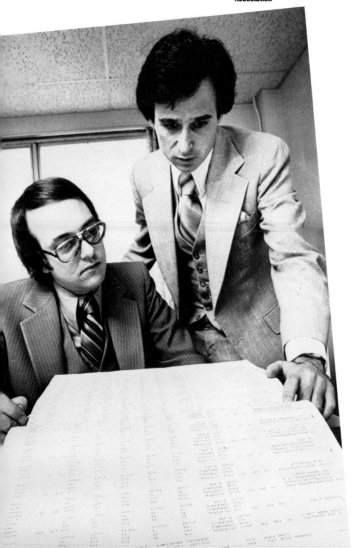

uninsured. In an attempt to alleviate a pressing problem, the cost of caring for those without insurance was to be spread among all payors, including Blue Cross; simply, insured patients would pay for hospital care for the poor. All rate recommendations were to be approved by the state Hospital Rate Setting Commission.

The purpose of the new system was to control hospital costs and to ensure financial solvency of hospitals. The policy was put forth in the first paragraph of what is known as Chapter 83 of public law: "It is hereby declared to be public policy of the state that hospitals and related health-care services of the highest quality, of demonstrated need, efficiently provided and properly utilized at a reasonable cost are of vital concern to the public health." The law also acknowledged issues that are still with us today—the need to "provide for the protection and promotion of the health of the inhabitants of the state, promote financial solvency of hospitals and similar healthcare facilities, and contain the rising cost of health services...."

The new system, based on Diagnostic Related Groups (DRGs), was considered revolutionary and a model for other states to follow. Hospitals were compensated a flat amount for a patient's care, based on an average for an illness and not on a per-diem rate as the SHARE system did. The DRG methodology assumed that patients suffering from similar diseases required similar hospital services at similar costs. Nonjustifiable costs above state-defined averages were not reimbursed; surpluses realized by below-average costs were retained by the hospital. DRG rates, like SHARE rates were set prospectively, subject to appeals and adjustments.

There were some 1,000 DRG categories. The costs of care were grouped into three categories. Direct Patient Care included nursing care, diagnostic and therapeutic ancillary services, hospital-based physician services, outpatient services, and some general services. Indirect Patient Care covered maintenance, general administration, utilities, and malpractice insurance. Capital Costs included depreciation, interest, leases, price-level adjustments, and property taxes.

While implementation of the DRG system was not due to be fully realized until 1980, Louis P. Scibetta, then executive vice president of NJHA, pinpointed some major problems with S-446 regulations in an August 1979 memo to CEOs of member institutions: "This system is completely untested and the impact on individual hospitals or the healthcare delivery system as a whole is not known...The proposed rate schedule (formula rate) will not include a factor for capital facilities allowance, legally mandated increases, Certificate of Need costs, or management costs. Any costs related to the above items must be pursued with the Commission. This means that as a practical matter every hospital will have to appeal."

Indeed, the appeal process was evoked by many hospitals. The Hospital Rate Setting Commission (HRSC) since 1978 has had jurisdiction over rates and appeals and is comprised of the Commissioners of Health and Insurance, two healthcare consumers, and a person experienced in hospital administration and finance. The commissioners serve ex officio; other members are appointed by the governor with advice and consent of the Senate for terms of four years.

In the appeals process, hospitals submitted uniform cost reports on their financial condition and operating characteristics, as well as a copy of each patient's medical record abstract and bill of charges. The Department of Health used this information to calculate that hospital's prospective payment rate and revenue budget. The Department of Health then proposed the payment rate to HRSC. A hospital then accepted or rejected the rate. An appeal process may have been invoked and required participation of the hospital, the Department of Health, an administrative law judge, the courts, and the HRSC.

Because the process of rate-setting was prospective, an end-of-year or final reconciliation was allowed. Year-end adjustments were made if actual experience differed from the projected experience. The value of the adjustment was reflected in the next year's payment rates and included interest penalties if a hospital overcollected on net patient-care revenue or interest payments if undercollection occurred.

Uncompensated Care Trust Fund Act

New Jersey guarantees all its residents access to hospital care, regardless of their ability to pay. Some states have county hospitals where care for those who cannot afford it is provided and subsidized by local taxes. But in New Jersey, general primary-care hospitals throughout the state serve both paying and nonpaying patients.

Providing care for the entire population, however, comes with a high price tag. Many citizens who earn too much to qualify for public programs such as Medicaid, cannot afford healthcare. And, each year, the number of work-

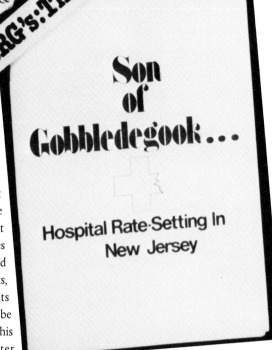

A 1976 NJHA publication focused on the confused state of setting hospital rates.
Courtesy, New Jersey Hospital Association

ing New Jerseyans without health insurance increases, either because they cannot afford it on their own or because their employer is not providing it as a benefit. Yet New Jersey hospitals continue to provide care for nonpaying patients—which added up to $710 million in 1991.

Beginning in 1987 when the Uncompensated Care Trust Fund Act was made law, hospitals were paid for uncompensated care—care for those who cannot or will not pay (including "bad debts")—by a surcharge of some 19 percent that was added to paying patients' bills.

The Trust Fund equalized the price for uncompensated care across hospitals. Some hospitals paid into the fund, while others received money from it. Without a fund, some hospitals would have had to mark up their bills only 2 percent, while others who care for more uninsured might have had to tack on a surcharge of 50 percent.

While many felt that the Uncompensated Care Trust Fund was not the most equitable means of paying for those who cannot pay, until a new funding source could be agreed to and implemented, the fund protected the state's hospitals from insolvency and made hospital care available to all who needed it.

The expiration of the Uncompensated Care Trust Fund in 1992 precipitated an overhaul of New Jersey's healthcare delivery system. NJHA supported broad-based funding on uncompensated care and was an active participant in the New Jersey Coalition of Health Care Reform, a group whose members included representatives of business, organized labor, the insurance industry, healthcare providers, and consumers—interest groups whose support was critical in making meaningful reform a reality for the state.

The Late 1980s —DRGs and Condition Critical

Across the state, hospitals experienced hardships in the late 1980s, brought on by New Jersey's tightly regulated hospital reimbursement system. Some 70 percent of hospitals regulated under Chapter 83 were financially ailing in 1988.

A number of environmental factors and unforeseen events precipitated the critical condition. Perhaps the most noticeable crisis of the late 1980s was a shortage of nurses, both nationwide and in New Jersey, where the average nurse vacancy rate was 17 percent. The "economic factor" component of hospital rates was not adequate to allow New Jersey to offer wages and salaries competitive with its neighboring states, Pennsylvania and New York. Nurses who normally

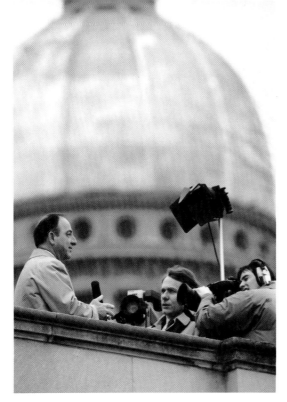

NJHA President Louis P. Scibetta holds an impromptu press conference at the Statehouse in Trenton to discuss the intricacies of a 1989 hospital payment rate issue.

Courtesy, New Jersey Hospital Association

Enormous expenses in research and development of "wonder drugs" are passed on to consumers, yet often they prevent even more expensive surgical intervention.

Photo by Rick Brady/Medichrome

would work in their home state were lured out of state by more attractive compensation packages.

While the cost of labor was the largest unanticipated factor in the financial ills of hospitals, several other crises occurred simultaneously, making the financial situation even worse. Increased regulation of medical waste disposal required millions of additional dollars to safeguard the environment. Another unforeseen event was the dramatic increase in the number of people with AIDS and the increase in the cost of their care. To protect healthcare workers from the spread of AIDS, the Centers for Disease Control recommended the institution of Universal Precautions in September 1987. Universal Precautions dictate the proper handling of patients' blood and other body fluids, syringes, and potentially infectious materials, adding still another cost item to hospitals' already burdened bottom lines.

Although New Jersey hospitals had achieved a level of cost efficiency unmatched by hospitals in other states, by 1988, years of cost containment left them in a critical financial condition. The state's hospital reimbursement system, mandated by law to meet hospitals' full financial requirements and keep them economically healthy, was failing. There was not enough built-in flexibility in the reimbursement system to make it responsive to unanticipated crises. In addition, the slowness of the state-run rate reconciliation process led to a situation where some hospitals were still seeking approval for rates for the previous five years.

The late 1980s saw some reimbursement reform that factored in adequacy for the unforeseen and saw the state sweeping clean prior rate-year adjustments, providing $1 billion in financial settlements to hospitals, to be paid over a three-year period. As hospitals entered the 1990s, for the first time in decades, a little breathing room was in the historically slim operating margins.

The 1990s and Beyond

On May 27, 1992, a federal court judge ruled that some patients did not have to pay the state-mandated hospital surcharge for uncompensated care. Judge Alfred M. Wolin found that the federal Employee Retirement and Income Security Act (ERISA), which prohibits states from regulating employee benefits, superseded the New Jersey state law and therefore, "forbids [self-funded] benefit plans from paying benefits for anyone other than a plan beneficiary." Self-funding is a common form of health insurance for employers with more than 200 employees. The people in a self-funded group, such as a union, pay into a fund that is for members of that group exclusively.

Because DRGs were based on the average statewide cost of treating patients with a similar diagnosis, the amount each patient was charged may have been higher or lower than the actual cost of care rendered. The surcharges to cover uncompensated care, which were added to the DRG rate, were ruled illegal.

If all this sounds confusing, it is. It was long the position of the New Jersey Hospital Association that it is unfair to charge some patients more than the actual cost of their care and some patients less. Hospitals in New Jersey advocated an alternative to the current hospital financing method.

In some ways, the federal ruling put New Jersey back to before 1968, to when the state could control only some payors and dealt with rate-setting the same as the rest of the country. But New Jersey has been a pioneer and an innovator under statewide legislation that set it apart from the rest of the nation. The Wolin ruling, which changed the all-payor status, allowed New Jersey to continue to lead the way and to serve as a spark to ignite the rest of the country in national reform of the healthcare financing system.

At the close of 1992, landmark legislation was passed in New Jersey. The Health Care Reform Act, a comprehensive and far-reaching piece of healthcare legislation, reformed the state's healthcare delivery system. The bill was designed to assure access to care for all, contain costs, promote consumer choices, encourage quality, make health insurance more accessible and affordable, and put clarity back into patients' hospital bills.

With this legislation, hospitals succeeded in replacing the confusing and complex DRG charges on patient bills with a new system that allows hospitals to bill patients for actual charges they incur. The legislation also substituted the 19 percent hospital bill surcharge to pay for care for the poor to a broad-based funding source by diverting money from the state Unemployment Insurance Trust Fund.

The New Jersey Hospital Association supported this new legislation, with various recommendations for amendments. NJHA plans to develop further legislation and regulation that will provide an orderly transition to a less regulated environment and to assure that hospitals that provide the most care in the toughest settings can get needed funds.

NJHA and its member hospitals have always been partners in contributing to reasonable and effective change. They will continue to work tirelessly to see that these meaningful reforms are put in place—and to assure that they work—for the good of all New Jersey hospitals and the people they serve.

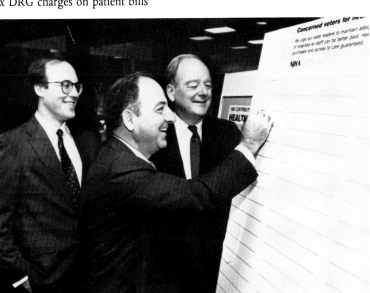

With rising costs of health insurance and an increase in treatment options, patients have become more informed healthcare consumers.
Photo by David M. Grossman

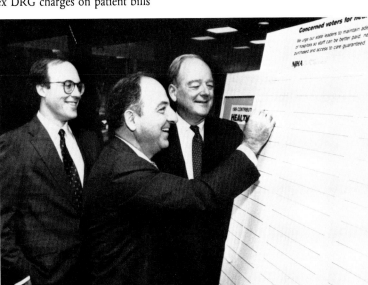

*A*long with more than 11,000 healthcare professionals, NJHA President Louis P. Scibetta signed a petition to help secure needed funding on behalf of NJHA's 112 member hospitals. Other association executives await their turn.
Courtesy, New Jersey Hospital Association

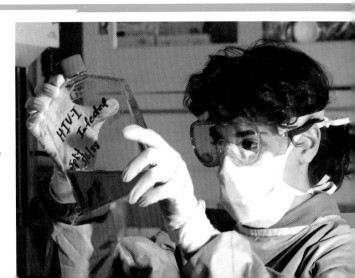

*G*iven the marvels of medical science in this century, the general public now expects miracle cures—for just about everything—to be discovered tomorrow.
Courtesy, New Jersey Hospital Association

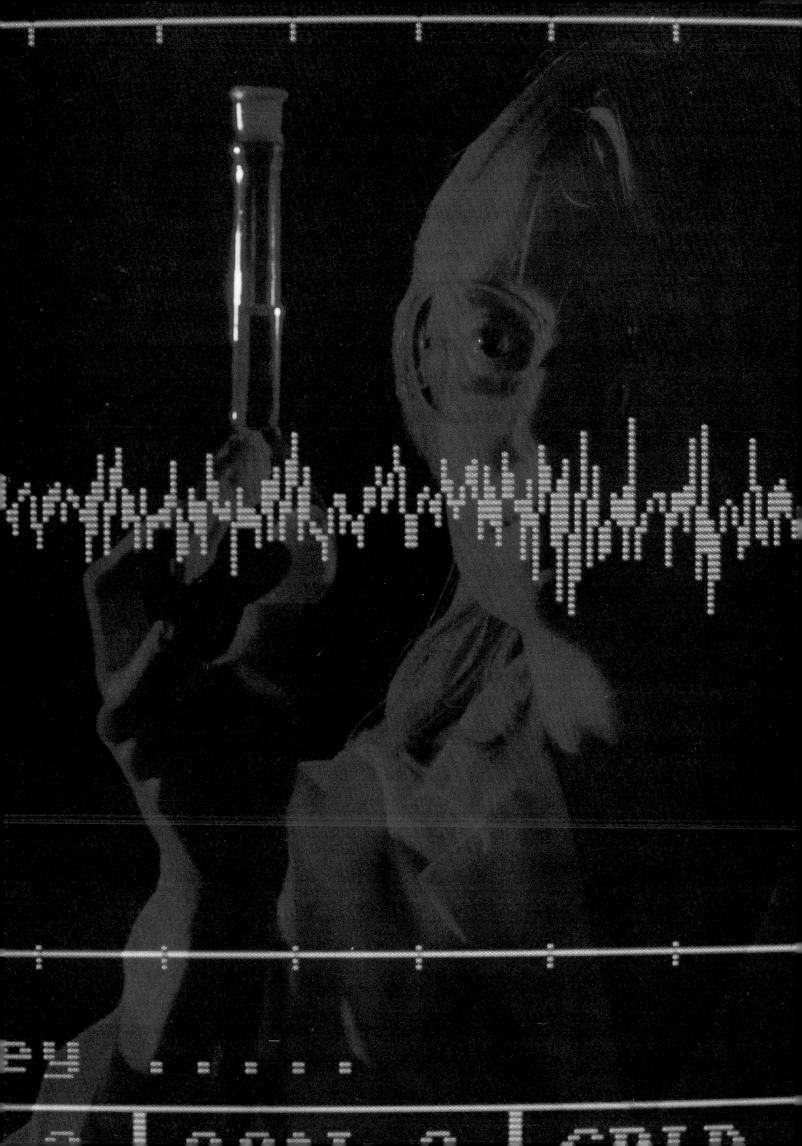

Many of New Jersey's healthcare "firsts" started with public and private enterprise—from dedicated individuals working in small university labs to multimillion-dollar Research and Development departments of giant corporations. These resources continue to revolutionize healthcare and support the vast needs of New Jersey hospitals.

The components of today's hospitals—physical facilities, equipment, medical procedures, management, and personnel—are supported by an immense network of products and services. The New Jersey Hospital Association and its member hospitals take advantage of New Jersey's geographic location, superior transportation systems, highly skilled labor pool, and diversity of industry.

Hospitals rely on relationships with educational institutions to train healthcare professionals and provide facilities for research. They need consulting services for legislation, legal and financial matters, ethics decisions, and administration. Their demands for quality products must be met. And, their long-standing interaction with insurers continues to be a foundation of contemporary hospital services.

As hospitals address social as well as medical issues, they expand into the community with more outpatient procedures and home care—all of which depend on products and personnel that the community provides.

Just as the past has been an extraordinary story of transformation, the future of healthcare and hospitals' vital role will also be remarkable. Legislative changes, continuing medical breakthroughs, innovative development of high-tech equipment, and specialized expertise are just a few trends that will affect healthcare.

The following pages introduce the organizations and institutions whose contributions have made this publication possible. Through affiliates such as these, the New Jersey Hospital Association remains at the forefront of reform and excellence in healthcare.

CHAPTER 10

PARTNERS IN PROGRESS

Healthcare Leaders
Support Innovation

The healthcare industry
has always benefited from
individuals and
organizations devoted to
finding ever-better
methods of healing.
Photo by Tom
Raymond/Medichrome

The New Jersey Hospital Association, founded in 1918, is a multifaceted organization whose synergy is fed by the 112 hospitals it represents, and whose objectives are critical to the healthcare industry and the well-being of New Jersey's 7 million residents.

Much has changed in 75 years, but then, as now, the mission of NJHA remains steadfast and clear: to be the advocate for New Jersey hospitals, their systems, and the healthcare services they provide.

Simple as it seems, that guiding principle entails a complex approach. New Jersey's acute-care hospitals, which operate on a nonprofit basis, are buffeted by fiscal constraints, bottom-line economics, the pressing health needs of society and its demand for top-flight care, the rapid development of technology and surgical techniques, and the strict regulatory climate.

The challenge for NJHA is to confront these issues, in order to develop and demonstrate responsible courses of action to prompt trust and confidence in New Jersey's hospital system, while providing day-to-day logistical support for members statewide.

Representing a $7 billion-a-year industry that employs more than 107,000, NJHA has evolved into a sophisticated, multi-tiered trade group.

Headquartered on a corporate campus in Princeton, New Jersey, NJHA's Center for Health Affairs is an administrative and tactical hub of issues-oriented management and advocacy, where the daily swirl of activities ranges from ordering supplies to lobbying legislators.

NJHA is directed by a board of trustees, which is advised by seven councils and each of their standing committees to sort, analyze, advocate, and initiate policy in the areas of auxiliary services, finance, government relations, planning, management practices, professional practice, and hospital governance.

Hospitals receive broad-based support through several NJHA-affiliated corporations based at the Center for Health Affairs, a facility available to the public for conferences, workshops, seminars, and meetings where more than 1,000 such gatherings are held each year.

The affiliated corporations offer research services and a multimedia library; insurance and employee benefit programs; a credit union and other low-cost financial services; and centralized group purchasing, medical record administration, and unemployment claims management, which help yield more efficient use of time, cost, and personnel for each individual hospital.

Communications is an increasingly critical area, and the NJHA staff is mobilized to educate the public through advocacy, forums, and lobbying activities. Maintaining this initiative is critical for NJHA in its continuing effort to assist the public and professionals in interpreting and grasping the fundamentals and complexities of the issues confronted by hospitals daily.

NJHA is recognized as one of the nation's premier hospital associations, a distinction earned through determined hard work, dedication to its members, and delivery of results.

As the 21st century draws near, NJHA remains committed to helping members plan for their futures by helping to shape public policy, containing costs, expanding the healthcare issues debate, and improving access to quality healthcare for all New Jerseyans.

NJHA's core services include advocacy, political action, health policy formation, and issues management. Here, as the association worked to represent hospitals' interests during intense labor reimbursement deliberations in 1988, NJHA President Louis P. Scibetta (left foreground) discusses strategy with member hospital CEOs at the Statehouse in Trenton.

Communication and education round out the list NJHA core services. The Smoke-Free Hospitals Program, among the first state hospital association sponsored campaigns to "clear the air" in health care facilities, symbolize the association's leadership in providing membership education and ongoing communication.

In the mid-1970s a medical malpractice insurance crisis gripped much of the nation. Claims and lawsuits had escalated dramatically, and hospital professional liability rates rose accordingly.

New Jersey's hospitals were seriously affected by the disruptions in the commercial insurance marketplace as some carriers withdrew because of heavy losses. To fill that void, a group of innovative hospitals implemented the Garden State's solution to the malpractice insurance crisis, creating an insurance organization in 1975 that would set the example for hospitals in other states to follow.

The organizational structure selected was that of an insurance reciprocal, to be called the Health Care Insurance Exchange (HCIE). Member hospitals, called subscribers, contributed the funds necessary to satisfy New Jersey's insurance standards and provide a margin of safety against catastrophic losses. The subscribing hospitals became insurers of each other through an attorney-in-fact, and were, in exchange, insured.

HCIE began writing professional and general liability insurance for hospitals in 1976. Within a year it had become the insurer of choice among the majority of hospitals in the state.

Toward the end of the 1970s it became clear that HCIE could enhance its value to its members by expanding coverages and services to help hospitals prevent incidents that would lead to insurance claims. Property and related coverages and a wide range of risk management and loss prevention services were added, the latter provided to policyholders at no additional charge.

Through the next decade HCIE expanded its product line to add workers' compensation, directors' and officers' liability, and excess insurance.

Princeton Insurance Company, a subsidiary, was established in 1982 to serve doctors and allied healthcare professionals. By the end of 1983 it insured 40 percent of New Jersey's physician market, and with HCIE ranked among the 20 largest medical malpractice insurers in the nation, according to data from A.M. Best, an organization that monitors and rates the nation's insurance industry.

Today Princeton Insurance Company provides professional liability coverage to thousands of medical and healthcare professionals throughout the mid-Atlantic region.

In 1991 the relationship between New Jersey's hospitals and HCIE was simplified by replacing the less-familiar structure of an insurance reciprocal with that of a stock company, called the Health Care Insurance Company, with New Jersey hospital policyholders becoming stockholders.

Its mission remains the same: to serve New Jersey's hospitals by providing dependable property and liability insurance coverage.

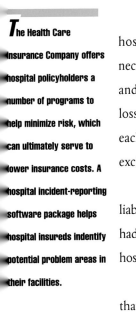

The Health Care Insurance Company offers hospital policyholders a number of programs to help minimize risk, which can ultimately serve to lower insurance costs. A hospital incident-reporting software package helps hospital insureds indentify potential problem areas in their facilities.

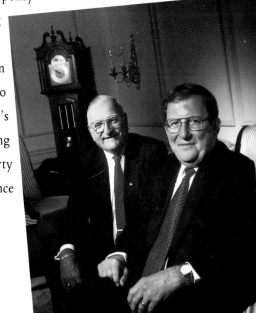

Barry D. Brown, chairman; and Donald E. Smith, president.

*I*t requires special people with special skills to handle the rigorous demands of an emergency department, including the split-second, life-saving decisions needed to stabilize and treat emergency department patients. In other words, the kind of people you find at Emergency Physician Associates (EPA).

Since 1978, this professional association of emergency physicians has given its client hospitals the highest levels of skilled, experienced, and dedicated emergency care. EPA offers staffing, management, and consulting services for the emergency department, house, and occupational health needs of their clients. EPA's programs are designed to improve patient care, promote cost efficiency, and enhance a hospital's standing in the community. This care is supported by an experienced management staff and complemented by support services and programs tailored to a hospital's needs.

Because the emergency department is often viewed as the front door of a hospital, it is imperative that the emergency department staff be top-notch professionals, up to the demands of their highly volatile work environment. EPA is synonymous with the very best. Their physicians are sensitive to the anxiety and trauma associated with emergency medicine and are skilled in ways to promote good patient relations.

EPA physicians treat more than 500,000 emergency patients annually at hospitals in the Middle Atlantic states. Their physicians work closely with the medical and nursing staffs, paramedics,

*E*mergency Physician Associates was founded in 1978 by James E. George, M.D., J.D., FACEP. George is the president and CEO of EPA, as well as a practicing emergency physician.

and ancillary staff of a hospital to provide the highest quality care. EPA physicians are specialists in the field of emergency medicine and lend their considerable talent, training, and expertise to their respective hospitals. In addition, EPA physicians are involved in teaching residents and medical students about the rigors and rewards of a career in emergency medicine.

Hospitals welcome EPA's contract management concept because they are confident in EPA's proven abilities. They look to EPA's specialized expertise to maximize the productivity of the department and positively influence the public's perception of their emergency department.

Founded by James E. George, M.D., J.D., FACEP, a practicing emergency physician and health law attorney, EPA understands that quality emergency services begin with quality physicians. EPA seeks out career-oriented physicians who meet high standards and adhere to the principles of the Joint Commission on the Accreditation of Healthcare Organizations and the American College of Emergency Physicians. Every physician's background, education, and experience is reviewed and presented to each client for their hospital credentialing purposes.

EPA encourages its physicians to pursue every opportunity for continuing medical education in order for them to be familiar with the latest developments, techniques, and technology in the dynamic field of emergency medicine. EPA sponsors educational

*E*PA physicians are ski... in providing quality eme... gency care to young an... old alike.

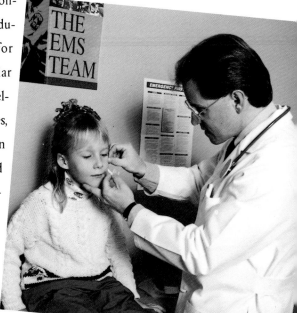

seminars and provides recertification courses in ACLS and PALS for the benefit of their physicians.

As further evidence of their commitment to continuing education, EPA publishes several national medical journals for emergency physicians and other healthcare professionals. These journals deal with topics such as emergency medicine, management of the emergency department, Total Quality Management (TQM) and Continuous Quality Improvement (CQI), malpractice, emergency nursing, and pre-hospital care.

EPA understands that its medical directors are the keystone of a successful emergency department. EPA routinely holds director workshops to further develop their directors' leadership, management, and administrative skills. Regular meetings are also held with the directors to review their emergency department's operation, and to monitor their progress in carrying out the client hospital's goals for the emergency department.

EPA has embraced the paradigms of Total Quality Management and Continuous Quality Improvement, and has developed a national reputation for its expertise in this important discipline. EPA has fostered a management philosophy that encourages teamwork, innovation, change, and communication, and is fully committed to implementing TQM/CQI at all of its client hospitals.

EPA's corporate staff devotes its broad-based resources to assisting client hospitals with marketing, billing, scheduling, and community relations. These efforts are directed toward achieving a positive public awareness of each hospital.

"EPA has always been a major contributor to emergency care in New Jersey and our region," says George. "We plan to continue our vital role in emergency care for many years to come."

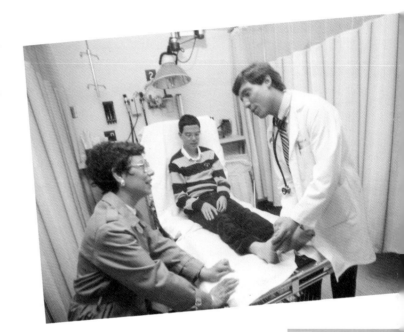

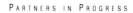

Johnson & Johnson is one of the most recognized names in the healthcare industry. With corporate headquarters in New Brunswick, New Jersey, and 1992 sales of $13.75 billion, Johnson & Johnson is the world's largest and most comprehensive manufacturer of healthcare products serving the consumer, pharmaceutical, and professional markets. In 1992 the company invested more than $1.1 billion in research and development. Johnson & Johnson has 168 operating companies in 53 countries, selling products in more than 150 countries. Today's work force of 84,900 worldwide is in stark contrast with the 14 employees who were with the company in the beginning, more than 100 years ago.

The company got its start in 1886 when three brothers, Robert Wood Johnson, James Wood Johnson, and Edward Mead Johnson, formed their own medical products company. Since the beginning, the company has been headquartered along the Raritan River in New Brunswick.

Under Robert Wood Johnson's leadership as president, the company joined physicians in the search for ways to fight disease and infection and became a leading healthcare company. James W. Johnson succeeded his brother and was president until 1932.

The early years were a time of expansion for Johnson & Johnson. Besides its early and rapid growth domestically, international growth of Johnson &

Johnson & Johnson's worldwide corporate headquarters, located in New Brunswick, New Jersey.

Johnson began in 1919 with the creation of a Canadian affiliate and was followed by the establishment of an affiliate in Great Britain in 1924.

The junior Robert Wood Johnson became the company's third president in 1932. During his tenure he wrote the Johnson & Johnson Credo, which describes the company's responsibilities to the people who use its products and services—customers, employees, communities, and stockholders. In addition, the corporate strategy of decentralization went into effect. This structure, which continues today under current chairman Ralph S. Larsen, allows each Johnson & Johnson company to have its own specialized mission and to operate with considerable autonomy.

The philosophy of decentralization is evident in the management of Johnson & Johnson, which divides its business into three sectors—consumer, pharmaceutical, and professional.

Consumer Companies

The consumer sector is Johnson & Johnson's largest. It consists of five major businesses: baby toiletries, sanitary protection, wound care, oral care, and over-the-counter drugs. A sampling of the consumer companies is included here.

JOHNSON'S Baby Powder and BAND-AID Brand Adhesive Bandages, sold by Johnson & Johnson Consumer Products, Inc., are well known consumer brands that have been industry leaders for decades. Considering the brief average lifespan of a consumer-branded product in the United States, it is remarkable that JOHNSON'S Baby Powder has been a leading product for more than 100 years. Other successful products include Johnson & Johnson Dental Floss,

Johnson & Johnson's decentralized structure allows its various companies to focus on products for specific markets.

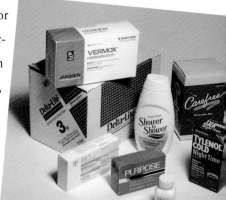

PURPOSE Soap and Moisturizer, and REACH and PREVENT toothbrushes. Another market leaders is Advanced Care Products, which in 1991 launched non-prescription MONISTAT 7, formerly the leading selling prescription product for vaginal yeast infections.

Personal Products Company is an excellent example of how Johnson & Johnson forms new businesses. Early on, the company was involved in the sanitary protection products business. This product line was so successful that it turned into the MODESS Division in 1933—now known as Personal Products. Today it provides a broad line of feminine hygiene products.

To increase its competitiveness in the over-the-counter medication business, the company has formed a joint venture with Merck & Co.—the Johnson & Johnson-Merck Consumer Pharmaceuticals Company.

McNeil Consumer Products Company, the leading manufacturer of over-the-counter analgesic products in the U.S., maintains market leadership with the TYLENOL acetaminophen line of products.

Pharmaceutical Companies

Johnson & Johnson has contributed to many advances in medicine since World War II. Today the pharmaceutical sector is the fastest-growing segment of the company's businesses.

Ortho Pharmaceutical Corporation is one of the oldest members of the Johnson & Johnson family of companies and one of the pharmaceutical operations highlighted here. Ortho began with one birth control product in the 1930s and is now a leader in prescription products for family planning. Its products include ORTHO NOVUM 7/7/7, the leading oral contraceptive prescribed by physicians in the U.S.

Ortho Diagnostic Systems Inc. and Ortho Biotech are spinoffs from the original Ortho. Ortho Diagnostic provides diagnostic reagents and instrument systems to hospital and commercial clinical laboratories and blood donor centers.

Ortho Biotech became a division in 1990. The company pioneered the first monoclonal antibody treatment and introduced PROCRIT (Epoetin alfa), a biotechnology-derived treatment for anemia.

In 1959 Johnson & Johnson acquired McNeil Laboratories, a concern noted for its sedation and muscle relaxant drugs. Now known as McNeil Pharmaceutical, it manufactures products like TYLENOL with Codeine—the leading prescribed narcotic analgesic.

Johnson & Johnson further strengthened its pharmaceutical business by acquiring the Belgian company, Janssen Pharmaceutica, in 1961. Janssen, a major source for pharmaceutical products, has introduced new drugs for use in fields such as anesthesiology, gastroenterology, immunology, cardiology, psychiatry, and oncology.

To reach more international markets, the company's Cilag Division, purchased in 1959, produces and distributes pharmaceutical products originated by other Johnson & Johnson companies.

Johnson & Johnson is at the forefront of many new challenging areas of medicine. R.W. Johnson Pharmaceutical Research Institute provides the pharmaceutical and diagnostic companies with innovative drug therapies. The Janssen Research Foundation Worldwide also conducts pharmaceutical

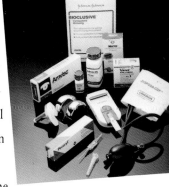

discovery and development in diverse areas. The company has established relationships with some of the world's leading research institutions such as the Scripps Institute and the James Black Foundation.

Professional Companies

The Johnson & Johnson name is visible in hospitals, physician offices, and clinics throughout the world, and healthcare professionals have come to depend on the company for bringing new technology-based healthcare products to market. A recent example of this innovation is the ACUVUE Disposable Contact Lens by Vistakon, which is among the professional sector companies.

Several of the professional companies focus on the needs of surgeons. Codman & Shurtleff, Inc., for instance, supplies surgeons and hospitals with surgical instruments, implants, disposables, and other products.

Ethicon Endo-Surgery helps surgeons develop new surgical procedures and the products that make small-incision surgery possible. The company manufactures a wide range of endoscopic instruments, internal and skin staplers, and ligation products. Ethicon Endo-Surgery was formerly a unit of Ethicon, Inc.—the world's leading manufacturer of sutures and related products for more than 100 years.

Other Johnson & Johnson professional franchises reach ophthalmologists, orthopedists, and interventional cardiologists and radiologists. Its Iolab Corporation markets ophthalmology products

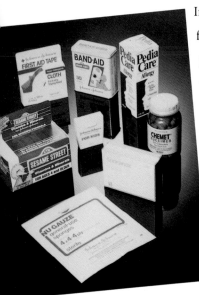

*T*he company manufactures a wide range of health-related products, like those pictured below.

including pharmaceuticals, intraocular lenses, microsurgical equipment, and instruments. Critikon, Inc., manufactures and markets cardiovascular monitoring and vascular access products. Orthopaedic products ranging from implants to bone fracture casting materials are manufactured by Johnson & Johnson Orthopaedics, Inc. Johnson & Johnson Interventional Systems Company provides interventional cardiologists and radiologists with products used in treating cardiovascular disease and related conditions.

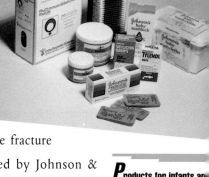

*P*roducts for infants and children, including those pictured above, are many and varied.

Johnson & Johnson Medical, Inc., provides healthcare professionals with products for wound management and infection prevention. These include disposable surgical packs and apparel, wound care sponges and dressings, sterilizing/disinfecting solutions, latex surgical and medical gloves, and topical absorbable hemostatic agents.

Johnson & Johnson Hospital Services Inc. develops and implements corporate marketing, customer service, and distribution programs on behalf of Johnson & Johnson professional companies. These programs respond to the needs of hospitals, multihospital systems, and distributors, to reduce costs and increase productivity.

Johnson & Johnson strives to serve the public interest by fulfilling the responsibilities stated in its credo. As the world's leading healthcare corporation, it is deeply committed to enhancing the quality of life for all of its constituencies. Besides producing products of high quality, the company seeks to conduct business in accord with the highest ethical standards.

erviceMaster, the national's largest provider of supportive management services to the healthcare industry, celebrated its 30th year of service in 1992.

In New Jersey, its employees have worked behind the scenes at scores of New Jersey hospitals for more than 25 years, applying their expertise in the areas of plant operations and maintenance, clinical equipment management, laundry and linen housekeeping, and food management services.

Today's economic climate requires hospital executives and their management teams to seize the most effective means of meeting their primary goals of quality and cost control. Variables in revenue, generation and reimbursement, patient mix, and utilization have created an urgent need for viable options to enhance the levels of service while holding operating expenses in check. A decline in the number of aggregate patient days can also aggravate the constant struggle to balance the books.

Increasingly, healthcare leaders are turning to ServiceMaster for the superior values offered by its specialized management of support functions and infrastructure. There is industry-wide recognition of the

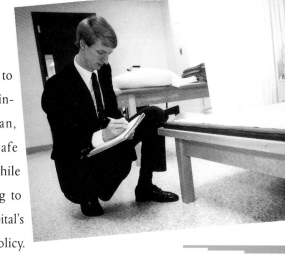

ServiceMaster professional management team, equipped to create and maintain a clean, healthy, and safe environment while strictly adhering to individual hospital's budgets and policy. ServiceMaster provides services to more than 1,300 healthcare facilities nationwide.

ServiceMaster is synonymous with strong management controls, high standards, and increased productivity, all of which assure consistent cost containment. Services in each hospital are customized for optimum performance and results.

Hospital administrators retain complete control of each service department, with ServiceMaster supplying the specialized management for that function, whether it be housekeeping, food services, or equipment maintenance. ServiceMaster offers a broad array of operational technical support services, ensuring plant safety, efficiency, and an uninterrupted flow of supplies.

The range of benefits is second to none; while ServiceMaster is tending to the day-to-day details, hospital administrators are free to turn their attention elsewhere.

ServiceMaster is happy to be a team player; it's what makes the company an integral and welcome component of hospital infrastructures nationwide.

*P*eace of mind comes from having a totally managed housekeeping department that continually strives to exceed your expectations.

*S*erviceMaster Food Management Services is dedicated to providing extraordinary food service to the New Jersey healthcare industry.

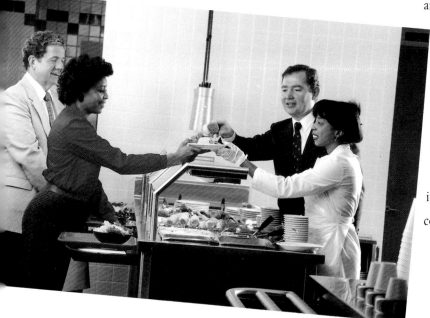

mmuno U.S., a subsidiary of Immuno International, is a leader in the field of biopharmaceuticals, with primary concentration on human plasma derivatives, vaccines, and diagnostics.

Immuno International is a corporate holding company comprising 20 subsidiaries located in Europe and Central and North America.

The Immuno Group has more than 30 years' experience on the cutting edge of plasma fractionation and vaccine development; worldwide, it employs more than 200 research scientists whose current emphasis is in the extraction of additional human plasma fractions and the development of new vaccines.

Its chief product groups are albumins, blood coagulation products, immunoglobulins, tissue adhesives, and vaccines. The most important disorders for which Immuno products are used include:

• Polytraumatic shock, where products rich in human albumin help to reestablish and improve blood circulation;

• Blood coagulation dis-

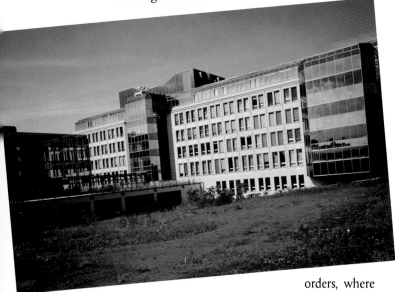

Immuno AG headquarters in Vienna, Austria.

orders, where products are used to replace missing blood coagulation capabilities;

• Short-term immediate immunization, using antibodies derived from human plasma for protection against infectious diseases;

• Wound healing and treatment, where adhesive materials produced from human plasma can effectively assist tissue and wound healing during surgery;

• Blood vessel obstruction, where a preparation obtained from plasma can be used for dispersing clots;

• Perinatology, where an anti-rhesus factor immunoglobulin prepared from human plasma helps avert rhesus factor incompatibility between mother and child. Another oral immunoglobulin lessens the risk of necrotizing enterocolitis in premature and newborn infants;

• Antibody deficiencies and autoimmune diseases, where an intravenous immunoglobin prevents bacterial infections in patients with low levels of gamma globulin;

• Long-term protective vaccination, where vaccines prepared from viruses or bacteria stimulate long-term protection.

The Immuno Group has more than 10 years' experience preparing vaccines against RNA viruses, the group to which AIDS-inducing viruses belong. In recent years a number of vaccines potentially active against AIDS have been developed, and extensive preclinical trials have been carried out on chimpanzees.

The first of these candidate vaccines are being evaluated in human patients, and are currently in Phase II clinical studies.

Immuno has other antiviral and antibacterial vaccines that are also in the preclinical or clinical trial stages.

Because the demand for currently available plasma products is growing steadily and will be difficult to fulfill in the future on the basis of human material alone, the production of certain plasma proteins using genetic engineering is a way of increasing avail-ability and may even provide alternatives to plasma derivatives or a way for improving the natural products.

Equally important to Immuno is the produc-tion of new vaccines, which it believes will provide products to treat diseases that until now have been untreatable, or for which treatment has not been suc-cessful, including certain disorders of blood circula-tion.

A third aspect of Immuno's research program is the study of severe, hospital-acquired infections, to which patients with extensive burns or other severe injuries are particularly susceptible. Products cur-rently being developed not only offer immediate prophylaxis, but are also important adjuncts to antibiot-ic therapy.

Immuno's strategy for the 1990s is to contin-ue intensive efforts in the field of genetic engineering. The aim is to develop innovative biological products that will be of prophylactic, therapeutic, or diagnostic importance.

This will extend the range and availability of plasma products beyond those based on raw materials, which will help to satisfy the growing demand for these items.

In all of its expanding activities, Immuno has never abandoned its special emphasis, thus lending its product range great coherence and creating a store of specialized scientific knowledge and technical know-how. This development strategy has not only been maintained in the company's research programs, but has also served as a guideline during the acquisition of new companies.

A number of new products, currently at an advanced stage of development, or on the verge of clin-ical trials, ensures that Immuno's current growth can be

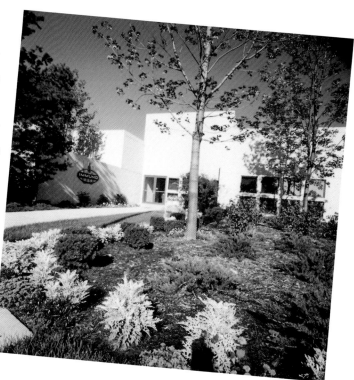

maintained during the coming years.

Immuno intends to remain loyal to core business, remaining committed to expand-ing its strengths in specialized markets.

Immuno-U.S., Inc., headquarters in Rochester, Michigan.

arre-National, Inc., and NMC Laboratories, subsidiaries of A.L. Laboratories of Fort Lee, New Jersey, manufacture specialty liquid and topical pharmaceuticals. By combining the resources and research capabilities of Barre and NMC, A.L. Laboratories has created a leading supplier of these specialty pharmaceuticals, raising the level of quality, distribution, and service.

Barre/NMC, which represents a combined 75 years' of experience in liquid and topical manufacturing, offers more than 170 different generic prescription and OTC products, including antibiotics, laxatives, psychotropics, and topical ointments, creams, and lotions.

Barre/NMC manufacturing facilities located in Baltimore, Maryland; Glendale, New York; and Lincolntown, North Carolina, combine to produce a full line of prescription and over-the-counter liquids and topicals. These specialty pharmaceutical products are packaged under the Barre label, the NMC label, and a broad range of private labels for chain drugstores and distributors.

Liquid pharmaceutical pilot plant assures product consistency from scientific development to full scale manufacturing.

In addition to retail drug chains, wholesalers, and distributors, Barre/NMC distributes products to hospitals, HMOs, and nursing homes, each of which takes advantage of the savings afforded by the purchase of generic products. Barre/NMC's average wholesale prices (AWP) offer substantial savings versus national brand name products.

Barre/NMC subjects its entire product line to strict quality assurance controls, standards that ensure

that precise guidelines are adhered to throughout the research and manufacturing process. From initial testing to regular sampling of batches for laboratory analyses, quality control is built into every step of the process. This scrutiny applies to the packaging, testing, and storage at each location, assuring high standards of safety, purity, and efficacy.

Positioned on the leading edge of technology, Barre/NMC is committed to quality and value. The company dedicates significant resources to research and development of its generic products years before brand-name patents expire.

Just as technology, research, and manufacturing are vital parts of the pharmaceutical business, so too is the timely delivery of products. Barre/NMC employs experienced sales and customer service specialists, who are backed up by the Electronic Data Interchange computer-linked network, which provides the latest electronic order processing, speeding the purchase and delivery of needed products.

As recognized specialists in liquid and topical pharmaceuticals, Barre/NMC will continue to utilize its research capabilities and scientific and manufacturing expertise to ensure its ability to provide superior products at low costs.

An advanced high speed tube filler fulfills custom needs by providing near 20,000 units per day.

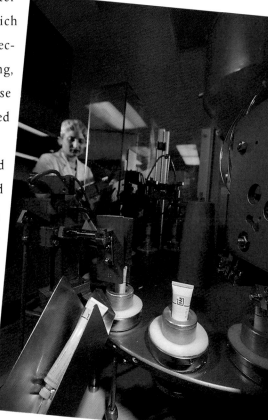

imes were tough when Henry Schein opened the doors of his corner pharmacy in 1930. The Great Depression had forced millions into the ranks of the unemployed. The nation's fledgling healthcare system could barely keep up with the demands being placed on it. There were no controls of any kind on the manufacture and distribution of pharmaceuticals to ensure their quality.

Yet, in this dismal picture, Henry Schein saw an opportunity to serve the needs of healthcare professionals by providing them with affordable pharmaceuticals of unquestionable quality. This vision has survived unaltered for six decades and has emerged as the central principle around which SCHEIN PHARMACEUTICAL has been forged.

In the five-year period between 1985 and 1990, the company increased its sales volume sixfold. In that same time frame expenditures on Research and Development grew seven times. That is the best measure of the SCHEIN PHARMACEUTICAL commitment to the future.

The company continues to develop strategies to maintain this commitment to excellence. SCHEIN PHARMACEUTICAL is determined to deliver the finest products to the emerging healthcare system of the future.

The strength of SCHEIN PHARMACEUTICAL in the American marketplace can be traced to two factors that set the company apart from its competitors.

The first is SCHEIN's manufacturing capability. Danbury Pharmacal, which comprises the company's solid dosage manufacturing facilities, has plants located in Carmel, New York, and Puerto Rico. These plants have been constructed to the most exacting specifications and have been equipped with the most advanced equipment and systems that are available.

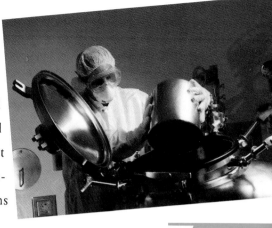

Taken at the Sterile Liquid Products Manufacturing Facility/ Phoenix, Arizona.

In Phoenix, Arizona, Steris Laboratories boasts a 125,000-square-foot manufacturing facility in which all of SCHEIN's sterile parenteral, ophthalmic, and otic products are produced. From initial formulation through inspection and packaging, only state-of-the-art equipment is used.

The second factor that sets SCHEIN PHARMACEUTICAL apart from other manufacturers is its people. At every level of the organization, company employees are dedicated to SCHEIN'S goal of providing healthcare professionals with affordable pharmaceuticals of unquestionable quality.

SCHEIN PHARMACEUTICAL has brought together a management team that brings experience and expertise while sharing Henry Schein's vision. The company's more than 1,000 dedicated people were chosen not only for their demonstrated abilities, but also for their ethical standards and professional commitment.

That's why SCHEIN is known for quick, correct answers, accurate orders, and swift deliveries. This commitment to customer service includes a 24-hour Drug and Medical Information Service Hotline to answer any technical or clinical query that a customer may have.

It is this dedication and commitment that will carry SCHEIN PHARMACEUTICAL on to its next 60 years of unparalleled success.

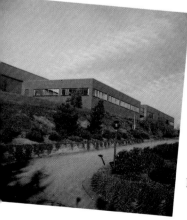

Solid Dosage Products Manufacturing Facility/ Carmel, New York.

National Westminster Bank NJ, New Jersey's fourth-largest bank, is a subsidiary of National Westminster Bancorp. It draws on the strength and expertise of the parent company, London-based National Westminster Bank PLC, one of the world's largest and strongest financial services organizations, with assets of more than $220 billion and offices in all of the world's major financial centers.

The bank has earned the trust and respect of its long-standing customers throughout New Jersey, including hospitals, healthcare centers, group practices, individual physicians, and other healthcare professionals.

Along with credit, NatWest NJ can offer cash management, access to financial and capital markets, and trust services to the businesses and professionals of New Jersey. These services are targeted to the specialized needs of hospitals and healthcare professionals. The bank always seeks to build and maintain long-term relationships with its healthcare industry customers.

Because hospitals today are increasingly focused on the bottom line, NatWest focuses on helping these institutions make optimum use of their cash flow.

The bank can assist hospital clients with everything from retirement plans to employee banking and on-site automated teller machines. Every customer is assigned a relationship manager who is able to provide complete, reliable, and continuous financial and business advice.

NatWest also customizes packages for physicians and other healthcare professionals to help finance a new or existing practice. The bank offers healthcare professionals lines of credit, mortgage financing, and even installment loans to provide cash for equipment and expansion. Healthcare professionals find that NatWest is eager to help them meet their financial goals right from the start of their careers. To this end, the bank offers financial seminars and advice to medical students and residents.

The personal financial needs of physicians and other healthcare professionals are met through a widely dispersed network of more than 130 branches throughout the state of New Jersey. Membership in the NYCE, CIRRUS, and MAC networks provides access to thousands of cash machines around the world. From MasterCard and VISA to home equity and student loans, NatWest NJ offers an extensive line of consumer credit products. In addition, personalized private banking services are available to high-net-worth individuals.

NatWest's strategy is to play to its strengths, keep its focus narrow, and concentrate on excellence in the quality of its products, personal service, reliability, and responsiveness. NatWest NJ provides hospital and healthcare professionals with a personal style of banking: relationship banking. After devoting considerable time to understanding customers' requirements, the bank gets closely involved with each customer, whether large or small, and considers itself a partner in each customer's financial success.

Drawing on assets of more than $220 billion, National Westminster Bank NJ focuses on building long-term personal customer relationships.

National Medical Rental Leasing & Sales, Inc. (NMI), supplies a wide range of infusion pumps, monitors, ventilators, incubators, and other critical-care products to a growing list of clients that includes The White House medical unit, Walter Reed Medical Center, managed healthcare systems, and corporate and industrial clients.

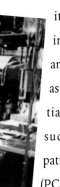

Critcal care ventilator therapy.

Its equipment performs vital tasks in a variety of settings, from a patient receiving bedside therapy at home, to critical-care units, operating rooms, and intensive-care units.

NMI provides technical assistance on all of its equipment, including intravenous, enteral, and ambulatory pumps, as well as pulse oximeters, sequential compression devices, suction equipment, and patient-controlled analgesia (PCA) pumps.

Quality assurance is synonymous with the equipment, service, and technical support provided by NMI. Hospitals and other clients are assured that their equipment has been thoroughly inspected to ensure functional integrity and electrical safety.

The equipment is delivered patient-ready. NMI purchases only new equipment, and before it is integrated into the NMI inventory it undergoes stringent evaluative testing to assure that it meets NMI guidelines for quality and is in compliance with manufacturers' specifications.

NMI has a computerized equipment-management system available to clients that can help track the utilization and status of all equipment in the hospital.

NMI utilizes a Rental Equipment Documentation program that adheres to hospital accreditation requirements, including a testing and labeling system that complies with JCAHO standards.

The Rental Equipment Documentation System Report includes inventory data associated with all rental equipment utilized by the hospital during a monthly reporting period, which significantly improves inventory control capabilities. Deliveries, on-site upkeep and maintenance visits, and repair and upgrade history are maintained by each hospital and NMI.

The NMI/Recall Modifications System is computerized to ensure incorporation of all manufacturer-required modifications. An extensive interactive system flags those units that require an upgrade, which ensures optimum performance from each piece of equipment.

Comprehensive documentation is an integral part of quality assurance with NMI, as is comprehensive in-service education, which is provided at the time of delivery and installation, and any time thereafter upon request. This service can be scheduled 24 hours a day to assure that all staff is given appropriate training.

In service of product lines.

NMI's comprehensive, exhaustive risk-management program is designed to minimize risk exposure for both the hospital client and NMI.

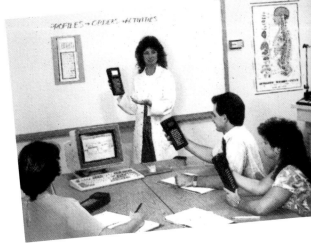

As society becomes more and more conscious of environmental issues, New Jersey hospitals are finding that being kind to their surroundings can mean saving money. Since 1977 GHR Consulting Services, Inc., an environmental and energy-management company, has provided savings to more than 40 hospitals in the state of New Jersey.

"Being experienced in all facets of environmental engineering and energy conservation, we're uniquely qualified to provide comprehensive and cost-effective solutions to the healthcare industry," says James Morrow, president of GHR.

In 1989 GHR was selected as the preferred contractor for environmental services by NJHA's Group Purchasing organization. GHR's full range of services includes site assessments, environmental permitting, hazardous waste management, underground storage tank management, regulatory planning, solid- and medical-waste management, air quality investigations, site remediation design, and more. Morrow identified waste management, underground storage-tank management and design, and regulatory compliance as the areas where hospitals most often benefit from GHR's expertise.

New and more strict environmental regulations have made it critical that hospitals work with a company that knows the regulatory ropes. Robert Roop, GHR's vice president of environmental services,

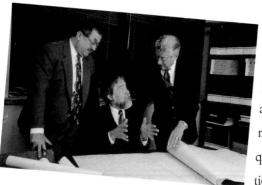

notes, "For many years we've been in constant contact with regulatory agencies. We have a good idea how these agencies will respond in specific instances and we are therefore in a very good position to negotiate with regulatory agencies on behalf of our clients."

An area of GHR's work in which regulatory considerations are of utmost importance is underground storage-tank management, and the design of upgraded or new systems. Federal and New Jersey laws have mandated that all tanks be upgraded to meet new standards. Underground storage-tank programs designed by GHR have helped numerous hospitals meet these standards, therefore saving a significant amount of money. When remediation is called for due to a compromise to the environment, GHR has the means and the experience to get the job done.

"Our years of work in solid-waste management and engineering have taught us that any hospital can benefit from a review of its waste-management practices," says Roop. Waste-management programs designed by GHR bring clients into regulatory compliance and often pay for themselves within a few years. Each hospital has different needs, and GHR can provide the full range of engineering and scientific expertise

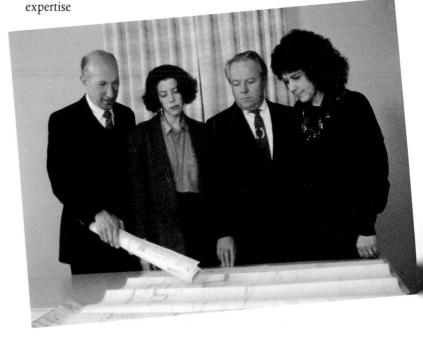

required, bringing to each job a global approach to problem solving.

Contracted to perform a waste-management practices audit for a division of a major New Jersey health system, GHR established the most cost effective waste-management option for the hospital group. "Our work with this client illustrates the many areas of expertise we bring to projects," says Roop. "We did audit work and analysis, instituted a recycling system, designed an incineration system, and assisted the hospital in obtaining permits." GHR continues to be the health system's consultant on all related environmental matters.

Energy management is the other side of GHR's business, and the company has been helping hospitals save money on energy bills since 1977. This effort has not gone unrecognized; GHR has achieved numerous energy-related awards, including the New Jersey Governor's Award for Energy Innovation and ASHRAE energy awards. Programs normally pay for themselves within three years or less, then continue to provide savings in the future.

The energy services offered by GHR include conservation opportunity analysis, the design of energy efficiency systems, construction management, program management, and computer-aided energy analysis. On behalf of its clients, GHR has arranged for government energy grants for the implementation of its recommendations.

Such was the case at one large New Jersey medical center, where GHR worked with the hospital to obtain more than $700,000 of Institutional Conservation Program (ICP) grants for systems that will bring the hospital energy savings of more than $500,000 per year. "Additionally, much of the equipment installed replaced systems that were near the end of their useful life. Thus the grant money paid one half of the replacement cost of equipment that was already budgeted for replacement," according to Morrow. "Further, the equipment we design often has lower maintenance costs and often provides a more comfortable work environment."

GHR's two areas of concentration, energy management and environmental engineering, are intrinsically linked in today's world.

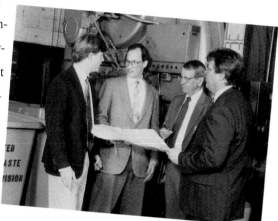

This is seen in the fact that energy efficiency is environmentally clean—it reduces carbon emissions, acid rain, and dependence on fossil fuels. This link is also seen in GHR's comprehensive environmental and energy-management planning.

On staff GHR has geologists; chemists; hydrogeologists; civil, mechanical, and electrical engineers; and has completed thousands of projects in 30 states. The company has performed work under the New Jersey Environmental Cleanup Responsibility Act, the Clean Air Act, the Clean Water Act, the Resource Conservation and Recovery Act, the Toxic Substances Control Act, the Comprehensive Environmental Response Compensation and Liability Act, and the Occupational Safety and Health Act.

As the preferred contractor for environmental consulting to the New Jersey Hospital Association, GHR looks forward to assisting in the valuable support that the NJHA provides to its membership in the years ahead.

GHR Engineers Alfred Lutz and Henry Nealis confer with Robert Davidson, Assistant Executive Director and James Grant, Director of Plant Services of West Jersey Hospital System. All of GHR's areas of expertise in environmental engineering and energy management were utilized in a multi-faceted project for the health care system.

SmithKline Beecham is one of the world's leading healthcare companies in pharmaceuticals, over-the-counter medicines, animal health, and clinical testing.

More than 300 SmithKline Beecham products are sold in more than 130 countries, with its strongest markets in the United States, Europe, and Japan.

Globally, SmithKline Beecham has two of the top 10 medicines—the antibiotic Augmentin, and Tagamet, a peptic ulcer treatment. Other prescription pharmaceuticals developed by SmithKline Beecham include the antibiotic Amoxil for treating common bacterial infections; Eminase, for treatment of heart attacks; Dyazide, for the control of hypertension; Engerix-B, a vaccine for the prevention of hepatitis-B; Paxil, for depression; and Relafen, for arthritis.

SmithKline Beecham U.S. headquarters: 1 Franklin Plaza, Philadelphia, Pennsylvania.

Popular consumer products include Aquafresh and Macleans toothpaste, the antacids Tums and Setlers, the Oxy acne treatment line, Massengill feminine hygiene products, Contac and Beecham's cold remedies, and Sucrets and N'ICE for coughs and sore throats.

With its United States headquarters in Philadelphia, SmithKline Beecham Pharmaceuticals concentrates its research and development in four therapeutic areas:

• Anti-infectives/biologicals, for treatment of bacterial, viral, and fungal infections;

• Cardiovascular, for treatment of heart disease and diseases of the circulatory system;

• Central nervous system, for treatment of anxiety, depression, compulsive and obsessive disorders;

• Inflammation and tissue repair, including treatment of arthritis.

Worldwide, the company invests nearly a billion dollars annually in research and development, with approximately 10 percent of its 54,000 employees involved in R&D.

Taking a tiny pill is a simple act, but the process of bringing it to market is a time-consuming, laborious task that involves the efforts of thousands of people and years of research, development, and clinical trials.

SmithKline Beecham has created specialist teams for each of the therapeutic areas in which it concentrates to streamline the pharmaceutical development process. These include the scientists who develop the drug in the laboratory, physicians who gauge its reaction and effectiveness on patients during clinical trials, and statisticians and regulatory affairs experts who ensure that the data collected during these studies will satisfy the exacting demands of the regulatory process.

SmithKline Beecham pharmaceutical products: To rate healthcare for New Jersey Hospital Association hospitals.

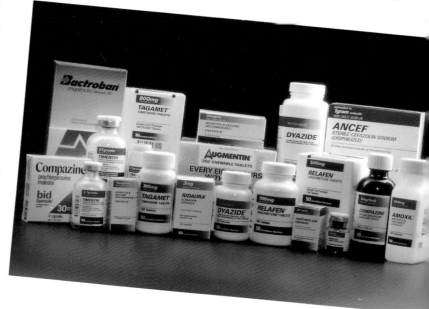

There are also patent attorneys, who protect the scientist's invention from being copied; market research and strategic marketing experts, who ensure that the product's profile matches the medical need; and clinicians, who demonstrate the product's effectiveness.

A process development, manufacturing, and quality assurance staff guarantees that the product can be manufactured to the highest standards on a consistent basis.

SmithKline Beecham aggressively pursues collaborative agreements with other healthcare companies and academic research facilities. This is a recognition that the pace of technological change and diverse sources of knowledge demand looking beyond its own R&D initiatives; augmenting its own efforts will ensure timely access to new product opportunities and emerging technologies, which will form the basis for new medicines.

The company supports major research programs at Johns Hopkins and Stanford University, and has its own venture capital company, SR One, Limited.

In 1985 SmithKline Beecham Pharmaceuticals became the first pharmaceutical company to establish a national accounts department to meet the growing needs of multi-hospital buying groups and managed care organizations.

SmithKline Beecham has worked with the New Jersey Hospital Association Group Purchasing

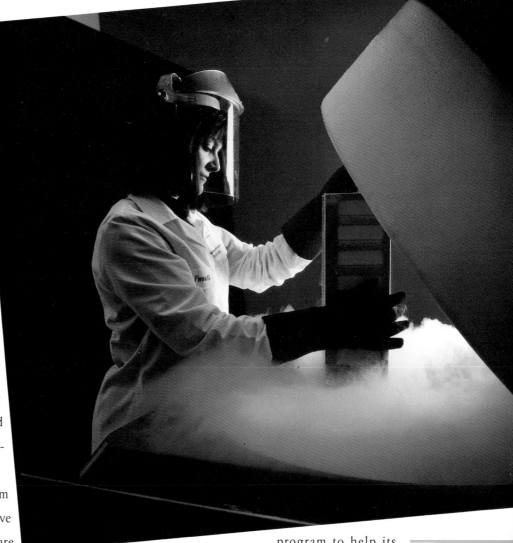

program to help its members control costs and improve the quality of their healthcare by providing top-rate pharmaceutical products at discounted prices. SmithKline Beecham has contracts with 24 multi-hospital groups in the United States; the NJHA Group Purchasing program is one of SmithKline Beecham's largest national accounts.

Research and development: thousands of SmithKline Beecham employees dedicated to discoveries for tomorrow's healthcare needs.

The company continues to grow, as does the National Accounts and Professional Relations department, which provides the infrastructure and support necessary to provide a complete contracting and management capability for business partners.

The National Accounts and Professional Relations initiative has proven its worth, building genuine, long-lasting business relationships that deliver savings on a portfolio of pharmaceuticals for large buying groups' member institutions.

With representation in more than 80 countries, Kabi Pharmacia is fast emerging as a world leader in the pharmaceutical industry. The 1990 merger of two Swedish-based pharmaceutical companies—Kabi and Pharmacia—formed this thriving multinational pharmaceutical corporation.

Dedicated to meeting the worldwide demands for new medicines, Kabi Pharmacia is at the forefront of research and development in products for eye surgery, growth disorders, cancer, inflammatory diseases, and thrombosis, and commands a leading position in clinical nutrition. The company currently produces or sells more than 400 pharmaceuticals used by hospitals and physicians around the world.

Pharmacia was founded in Sweden in 1911 and established its United States subsidiary in 1948. Pharmacia's headquarters in Piscataway, New Jersey, remains the U.S. headquarters for Kabi Pharmacia.

Shortly after the 1950 launch of Azulfidine® for treatment of ulcerative colitis, the company gained national recognizition for the marketing of major pharamaceuticals in the United States. Still widely prescribed, Azulfidine®, Azulfidine En-tabs®, and Dipentum® give Kabi Pharmacia its prominent role in treating gastroenterologic disorders. Pharmacia made significant strides in ophthalmic surgery with the development of Healon®, a substance that protects eye tissue during surgical procedures and enhances tissue compatibility.

Kabi became renowned for its achievements in biomedical and genetic engineering. A 60-year-old tradition of aggressive medical research and a series of mergers and acquisitions have contributed to a strong pharmaceutical presence worldwide. For example, Kabi revolutionized intravenous nutrition with the development of Intralipid®, the first safe fat emulsion for intra-

venous use. It has become the international standard and is unsurpassed in terms of documented use in millions of treatment situations.

Kabi Pharmacia's success evolves from innovative research strategies, optimization of resources, marketing expertise, and keen foresight into the ever-changing needs of the medical community.

Meeting the needs of test laboratories, Kabi Pharmacia's diagnostics division specializes in the areas of infectious diseases and the in-vitro allergy diagnosis markets and dominates the market in both Europe and Japan.

Research is a major function of all Kabi Pharmacia's business units. Dedicated solely to the development of pharmaceuticals, the company invests nearly one-sixth of its income into research. Its operating companies maximize these efforts

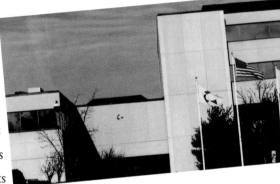

The U.S. headquarters Kabi Pharmacia, Inc., in Piscataway, New Jersey

by focusing on sharing resources and avoiding duplication of effort.

Kabi Pharmacia's worldwide presence is represented by some 11,000 employees in 30 plants in 20 countries, whose common goal is to be an international, research-intensive pharmaceutical company devoted to anticipating and adapting to new conditions and opportunities in the healthcare industry.

With a deep commitment to transforming research results into effective, cost-efficient pharmaceuticals, Kabi Pharmacia plans to use its strength in medical innovation, market intelligence, and extensive research efforts to firmly establish a dominant marketing position in the United States, Europe, and Japan.

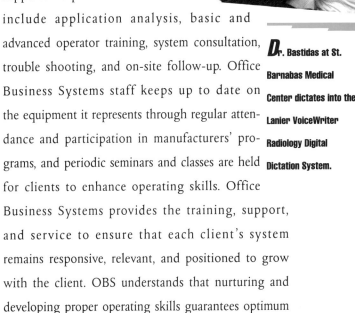

Adapting technology to fit the specific needs of its clients, Office Business Systems (OBS), Inc., provides custom-designed, quality products to increase productivity in the workplace.

Office Business Systems is the oldest and largest distributor of full-line office automation systems in New Jersey and is an exclusive representative of Lanier Voice Products. For 60 years Lanier has offered solutions to healthcare professionals and is a leader in hospital automation. Lanier provides the total solution to the healthcare reporting needs. Components of the total solution are digital dictation, medical transcription systems, chart tracking and deficiency systems, and optical chart storage and retrieval systems.

Founded in 1965, OBS has continued to evolve as new technology is introduced into the marketplace and the demands of its clients grow more sophisticated. It has a broad client base in the legal, medical, hospital, educational, and emergency-response markets.

As a demand for information and communication increases, Office Business Systems and Lanier continue to meet that demand. By providing state-of-the-art systems to New Jersey hospitals, Office Business Systems, teamed with Lanier, has become the unsurpassed leader in its field.

Because no two applications are the same, Office Business Systems is geared to adapt the technology to satisfy the specific need of the customer's office environment, whether it be the hospital that needs specialized records faxed from one department to another or a police department's 911 emergency dispatch system.

The Medical Records at Hackensack Medical Center utilizes Lanier's Medword Transcription System and VoiceWriter Digital Dictation System.

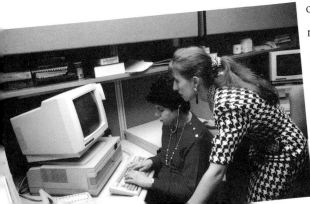

OBS marketing support representatives provide unparalleled pre-sale and post-installation support. Responsibilities include application analysis, basic and advanced operator training, system consultation, trouble shooting, and on-site follow-up. Office Business Systems staff keeps up to date on the equipment it represents through regular attendance and participation in manufacturers' programs, and periodic seminars and classes are held for clients to enhance operating skills. Office Business Systems provides the training, support, and service to ensure that each client's system remains responsive, relevant, and positioned to grow with the client. OBS understands that nurturing and developing proper operating skills guarantees optimum results for the client.

Dr. Bastidas at St. Barnabas Medical Center dictates into the Lanier VoiceWriter Radiology Digital Dictation System.

Technicians in the OBS service department represent more than 260 years of experience. OBS field engineers are highly trained and skilled in all areas of equipment and systems maintenance. Staffing and ongoing training is specifically focused on each product division.

OBS technicians and engineers are backed by a computerized inventory tracking system, and the installation department makes on-site surveys to ensure accurate estimates for each installation or relocation of equipment.

OBS has earned its reputation for quality, top-flight service by anticipating and responding to clients' particular needs. Backed by trained specialists and the latest, most advanced equipment in the marketplace, OBS' communications superiority will continue to assure its clients a competitive edge.

oechst-Roussel Pharmaceuticals, an affiliate of Hoescht AG, one of the top five pharmaceutical companies in sales worldwide, is committed to discovering, developing, and manufacturing innovative prescription drugs to meet current and future needs of healthcare professionals in treating illness and improving patients' quality of life.

Headquartered in Somerville, New Jersey, the company is part of the Life Sciences Group of Hoechst Celanese Corp., a wholly owned subsidiary of Hoechst AG of Germany.

Hoechst-Roussel's manufacturing, sales, and marketing activities are centered at the Somerville complex, but the primary thrust is research and development in the neurosciences. The Hoechst-Roussel Clinical Research Department works on new compounds for the treatment of Alzheimer's disease, schizophrenia, and obsessive-compulsive disorders.

Hoechst-Roussel's $20-million, 46,000-square-foot molecular neurobiology laboratory at the Somerville complex is expected to open in 1993. The three-story structure will expand Hoechst-Roussel's capabilities for finding treatments for Alzheimer's and other neurological disorders.

Typically, researchers at the facility have about 25 new drug candidates under development, including antibiotics, antihypertensives, anti-diabetes, and hemorheologic agents. HRPI enlists the aid of New Jersey hospitals, including Robert Wood Johnson University Hospital and St. Joseph's Medical Center, for clinical trials of its products.

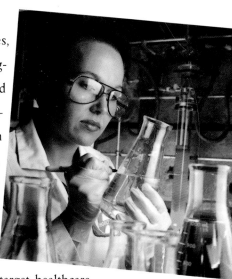

The major products of Hoechst-Roussel are prescription drugs. Sales efforts target healthcare professionals in physicians' offices, pharmacies, and hospitals. The firm's 800-member field sales force is supported by nine regional offices, which include a team of specialists with doctorates in the biological sciences who provide state-of-the-art technical information, plus specialists in government affairs, managed healthcare systems, and national hospital accounts.

A major segment of the sales effort is directed at hospital buying groups, which maximizes volume sales of Hoechst-Roussel products to members of the buying consortiums.

Among the leading Hoechst-Roussel prescription drugs are Claforan® (cefotaxime sodium), a cephalosporin antibiotic used to treat serious infections; Trental® (pentoxifylline), a hemorheologic agent used to improve blood flow and treat intermittent claudication, a symptom of peripheral arterial disease; and DiaBeta® (glyburide), an oral hypoglycemic agent used in the treatment of non-insulin-dependent diabetes.

Other products include Altace® (ramipril), an ACE-inhibitor used in the treatment of hypertension; Prokine® (sargramostim), GM-CSF, a cykotine used with bone marrow transplantation; Lasix® (furosemide), a diutetic used in the treatment of congestive heart failure; Topicort® (desoximetasone), a topical corticosteroid;

Dr. Gregory Shutske, principal research scientist, Chemical Research, and Michael Cornfeldt, associate directors, Biological Research, examine a rendering of the brain at the Hoechst-Roussel Pharmaceuticals Inc., laboratories in Somerville, New Jersey. Both are members of a team of scientists who are developing compounds to treat Alzheimer's disease.

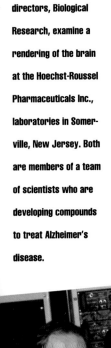

A researcher at Hoechst-Roussel Pharmaceuticals purifies potential drugs for Alzheimer's disease by column chromatography, the physical separation of organic compounds.

and Loprox® (ciclopiroxolamine), a topical antifungal.

Hoechst-Roussel Pharmaceuticals is an outgrowth of the merger of two companies. In 1960 Hoechst AG acquired Cincinnati-based Lloyd Brothers, Inc., which was founded in 1873 by pharmacist John Uri Lloyd, a prolific researcher of drugs derived from plants. Six years later the company became known as Hoechst Pharmaceuticals Company.

In 1974 Hoechst AG acquired a majority stake in the French research and chemical firm, Roussel Uclaf. Hoechst then combined the U.S. Hoechst Pharmaceuticals with Roussel Uclaf's pharmaceutical interest in the United States to form Hoechst-Roussel Pharmaceuticals Inc.

The parent company, Hoechst AG, was created in 1863 and has grown into one of the world's largest and most progressive chemical and pharmaceutical manufacturers. It operates more than 250 companies in 120 countries, employing more than 170,000 people. It spends more than $2 million each working day on pharmaceutical research. Worldwide, company sales exceed $28 billion annually, with pharmaceutical sales representing nearly 20 percent of that total.

In 1987 Hoechst acquired Celanese Corporation, forming Hoechst Celanese Corporation, one of the largest companies in America. Hoechst-Roussel is a subsidiary of that corporation.

In addition to pharmaceuticals, the Hoechst worldwide family of companies is involved in the development, manufacture, and sales of chemicals, dyestuffs, synthetic fibers, films, diagnostic equipment and reagents, fertilizers, plastics, herbicides, food additives, and products for animal health.

The management philosophy of Hoechst-Roussel embraces the wisdom and tradition of the parent company, recognizing that its people are its most important asset. Innovation, leadership, and personal and professional growth are encouraged and rewarded.

Employees are consistently challenged to maximize each individual's potential; there is an ongoing effort to direct the decision-making process down into the organization, to let the people that are doing the job run the activity.

That same level of energy and commitment is directed toward the surrounding community. Recognizing the need for American students to be competitive in the global community, Hoechst-Roussel and Hoescht Celanese contribute significant resources and personnel for a variety of programs with area schools and national universities.

Hoechst-Roussel sponsors summer fellowships for teachers; chemistry achievement rewards for graduating seniors; laboratory tours; and internships for pharmacy students and college seniors. Hoechst-Roussel also donates excess equipment and glassware to area schools and colleges, including Rutgers University.

A researcher at Hoechst-Roussel Pharmaceuticals, Inc., in Somerville, New Jersey, performs a receptor binding assay for analyzing the interaction of potential drugs for Alzheimer's disease with neurotransmitter receptors.

*F*riederike Wirtz-Brugger, Research Pharmacologist for Hoechst-Roussel Pharmaceuticals Inc., maps brain waves on an electroencephalograph for research on Alzheimer's disease.

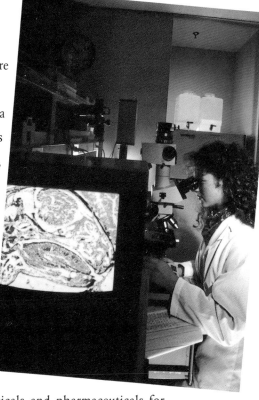

Schering-Plough Corporation is a worldwide, research-based company that discovers, develops, manufactures, and markets pharmaceutical and healthcare products. A highly competitive market leader, Schering-Plough sales reached $3.62 billion in 1991. A leader in the pharmaceutical industry, the company has more than 20,000 employees serving the health and personal care needs of people throughout the world.

Schering's ties to New Jersey began in 1934 when its first research building was opened in Bloomfield. Today the company has several facilities in New Jersey at Madison, Liberty Corner, Kenilworth, Union, and Lafayette. Madison is the site of Schering-Plough corporate headquarters, and Liberty Corner is headquarters for Schering-Plough HealthCare Products, the company's over-the-counter unit. The company's Safety Evaluation Center, where new pharmaceutical compounds are tested, is located in Lafayette.

Schering-Plough commitment to research is especially evident in Kenilworth, the site of the company's new $300-million pharmaceutical discovery center. Kenilworth is also a major manufacturing site, as well as headquarters for Schering-Plough International, which markets prescription pharmaceutical and over-the-counter products in more than 125 countries.

At Union, a wide array of products is manufactured, packaged, and distributed to customers. Union is also the site of a biotechnology group, as well as headquarters for Schering-Plough Animal Health, which develops and markets worldwide a broad range of biologicals and pharmaceuticals for animals.

The discovery and development of innovative pharmaceuticals is key to Schering-Plough's success. Committed to growth through research, the company has invested nearly $3 billion in research and development since 1980.

With 2,500 scientists and researchers worldwide, New Jersey laboratories; the DNAX Research Institute in Palo Alto, California; and biotechnology facilities in Dardilly, France, and Brinny, Ireland, the company has been a pioneer in immunology and

Schering-Plough's new, $300-million pharmaceutical discovery center, Kenilworth, New Jersey.

Committed to growth through research, the company has invested nearly $3 billion in research and development since 1980.

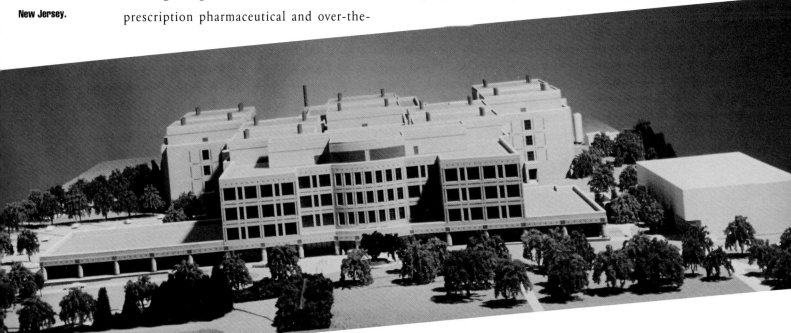

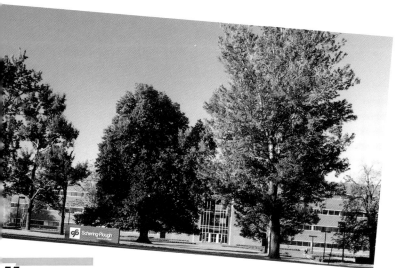

biotechnology research. In fact, Schering-Plough is a leading biotechnology company with biological products being marketed worldwide.

Schering-Plough Pharmaceuticals

Schering-Plough Pharmaceuticals—an operating unit of Schering-Plough Corporation—accounts for 75 percent of the company's sales. Employing state-of-the-art manufacturing and stringent quality-control techniques, this unit manufactures and markets prescription pharmaceuticals under its Schering Corporation and Key Pharmaceuticals labels. Major pharmaceuticals include respiratory products, dermatologicals, anti-infectives, and cardiovasculars.

Schering-Plough Pharmaceuticals also manufactures and markets superior contact lenses through its vision care business, Wesley-Jessen, headquartered in Chicago.

Schering-Plough HealthCare Products

Capitalizing on the reputation of such popular brand names as AFRIN®, DRIXORAL®, TINACTIN®, CORRECTOL®, DR. SCHOLL's®, and COPPERTONE®, Schering-Plough HealthCare Products—another operating unit of Schering-Plough

Corporation also based in New Jersey—is building its position as the leading manufacturer and marketer of a broad range of over-the-counter pharmaceutical and personal care products.

Schering-Plough holds a unique position as the nation's premier company in switching prescription products to OTC status, having gained market clearance for eight such products to date.

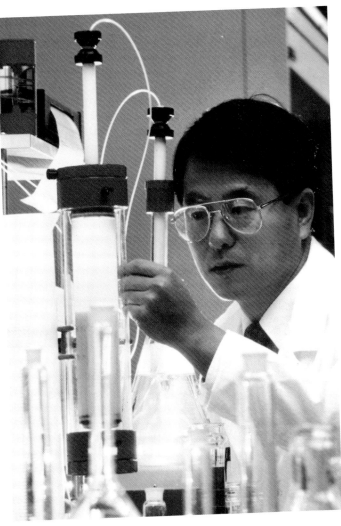

I n 1992 the achievement list at UMDNJ was topped by two major items—the passage of the University Flexibility Act of 1992, which greatly enhances UMDNJ's independence and operating flexibility, and the approval of the UMDNJ-School of Nursing.

These advances are propelling UMDNJ into a new era of service to the people of New Jersey. Together they mark another turning point in the brief but enterprising history of the state's university of the health sciences.

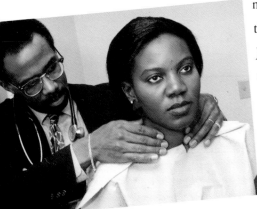

It was little more than 22 years ago that Dr. Stanley S. Bergen, Jr., became the institution's first president, having accepted the challenge of creating a statewide system of health-sciences education, basic and clinical research, and healthcare services.

Dr. Bergen proved to be a master architect. Starting in 1971 with the state's fledgling medical and dental schools, he crafted the nation's largest university devoted solely to the health sciences.

Today the University of Medicine and Dentistry of New Jersey consists of three medical schools, a dental school, a nursing school, a graduate school of biomedical sciences, and a school of health-related professions at campuses in Newark, Piscataway/New Brunswick, Stratford, and Camden. More than 4,500 students and 10,000 employees are based at the four campuses.

The UMDNJ-School of Nursing—the institution's seventh school—offers a career-ladder curriculum

Dr. Mark Johnson, chairman of the Department of Family Medicine at UMDNJ-New Jersey Medical School, examines a patient.

with programs leading to degrees at the associate, bachelor's, and master's levels. The A.S. and B.S. programs are offered jointly with Middlesex County College and Ramapo College of New Jersey, respectively.

In addition, the university has developed a comprehensive healthcare system providing New Jerseyans with state-of-the-art care delivered through its four core teaching hospitals, two community mental health centers, and more than 100 affiliated hospitals and other healthcare agencies.

The community-based healthcare and outreach services offered by UMDNJ's affiliate hospitals, clinics, and outreach programs form a statewide safety net for underserved and underinsured citizens of New Jersey. These include:

• UMDNJ-University Hospital, Newark, offers one of the nation's most comprehensive programs of primary care through diverse outpatient programs. The hospital also offers Kid Care, a mobile service for children at city housing projects and homeless shelters.

• The Chandler Health Center, New Brunswick, operated by UMDNJ-Robert Wood Johnson Medical School, serves some 10,000 area residents. It houses one of the state's largest Women, Infants, and Children (WIC) programs, and is a site for HealthStart, which reduces infant mortality through home visits and counseling.

• In the Camden area, extensive community services to the needy are offered by the UMDNJ-School of Osteopathic Medicine and UMDNJ-Robert Wood Johnson Medical School at Camden and their affiliate hospitals.

• The UMDNJ-New Jersey Dental School, Newark, is establishing a network of community oral healthcare services that provide dental treatment

Dr. Stanley S. Bergen, Jr., president of UMDNJ.

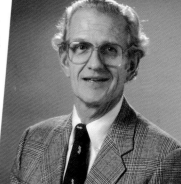

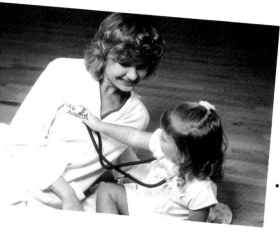

and education to needy populations statewide.

• UMDNJ's Community Mental Health Centers in Newark and Piscataway offer comprehensive individual and group services to children, adolescents, and adults.

The university has also developed leading research programs, gaining national attention for studies into such areas as AIDS, tuberculosis, and Parkinson's disease. In 1992 UMDNJ's programs in research and education were supported by more than $100 million in federal, state, and private funds.

UMDNJ's impact on the well being of New Jerseyans is compelling:

• One in four practicing physicians in the state is affiliated with UMDNJ. Of the 16,000 licensed physicians, 4,500 are either a graduate, faculty member, or postgraduate physician in a UMDNJ-sponsored residency program.

• Of the 6,000 dentists practicing in the state, 1,300— more than one in five—is a UMDNJ graduate or faculty member.

• Of New Jersey's 119 hospitals, 87 have affiliation agreements with the university.

Beyond its missions of education, research, and patient care, UMDNJ is a major force in the state's economy. In 1991 UMDNJ received $254 million in state support. Yet for every state dollar, UMDNJ attracted another $1.50 from nonstate sources. As a result UMDNJ returned some $635 million to the economy.

UMDNJ's extraordinary growth over the past two decades is a tribute to its tireless president. A week after he arrived in July 1971—just months after the institution was created by the State Legislature—ground was broken for the $250-million Newark campus.

In the ensuing years the university mushroomed, expanding to four campuses. To name just a few of the milestones, UMDNJ:

• Attained status in 1981 as New Jersey's second state university (Rutgers University was the first);

• Emerged as a national leader in recruiting, retaining, and graduating minority students in medicine and dentistry, and in recruiting minority faculty members;

• Established, in partnership with Rutgers, the Center for Advanced Biotechnology and Medicine (CABM) and the Environmental and Occupational Health Sciences Institute (EOHSI).

The university moved into a new era with passage of the University Flexibility Act of 1992. This law empowers UMDNJ to form partnerships with private industry, paving the way for new joint research and healthcare ventures, especially with New Jersey's vast pharmaceutical industry.

As Governor Jim Florio said when he signed the legislation into law: "This bill puts UMDNJ on equal footing with the health-science universities in other states when it comes to capturing research dollars. These public-private partnerships will fuel the new business ventures of the twenty-first century and keep healthcare and pharmaceutical jobs here in New Jersey."

Through this new legislation, and through its unwavering goal of providing New Jersey with the latest and most innovative healthcare programs, UMDNJ stands ready to meet the healthcare challenges of this decade and beyond.

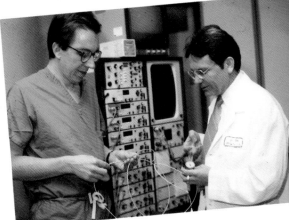

arner-Lambert traces its beginnings to the early 1850s. A multinational company, it is devoted to developing, manufacturing, and marketing quality healthcare and consumer products. It employs 35,000 people in more than 130 countries, including 3,000 at its corporate headquarters site in Morris Plains, New Jersey.

The company now ranks among the top 14 pharmaceutical companies worldwide. It is the ninth-largest pharmaceutical company in the U.S.

Warner-Lambert's pharmaceutical products are marketed under the Parke-Davis and Warner Chilcott names. More than 300 branded and generic products are available for the treatment of numerous major medical conditions.

Innovative research has long been a driving force at Warner-Lambert, with more than 2,000 scientists and technicians working at 10 major laboratories worldwide, including the Morris Plains facility. The company concentrates its pharmaceutical research efforts in three major therapeutic areas, which are cardiovascular disease; chemotherapy, including anticancer and anti-infective treatments; and central nervous system disorders.

A substantial portion of the Parke-Davis pharmaceutical discovery and development effort is directed at the management of cardiovascular disease. Current scientific activity spans all cardiovascular risk factors. Parke-Davis pharmaceutical products are used to treat cardiac arrhythmia,

Pictured here are some of the company's advanced systems for discovering and developing compounds for the treatment of diseases related to the central nervous system (CNS). CNS research is among the highest scientific priorities for Warner-Lambert.

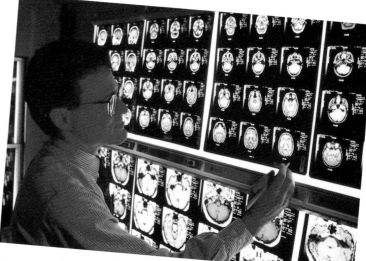

hypertension, and ischemic heart disease, as well as to aid the regulation of blood lipids.

Parke-Davis has had a pioneering role in the prevention of coronary artery disease. Its lipid-regulating Lopid was the first drug proven to reduce cardiovascular disease risk. Lopid is among Parke-Davis' most successful products.

Parke-Davis has become a growing force in the treatment of hypertension through the ACE-inhibitor Accupril. The company's impact on cardiovascular health has also been expanded by the recent introduction of the Nicotrol transdermal nicotine patch. This aid to smoking cessation offers significant patient advantages.

Parke-Davis has held a leadership position in central nervous system (CNS) disease since its development of Dilantin more than a half-century ago. Dilantin remains the leading treatment for epilepsy. Committed to an active drug research program in the CNS area, Parke-Davis is pressing ahead with development of new drugs for the treatment of Alzheimer's disease.

In addition to pharmaceuticals, Warner-Lambert manufactures and markets a broad range of over-the-counter pharmaceuticals; healthcare-related

The company works intimately with a number of leading teaching hospitals in the clinical evaluation CNS and other drugs. Among the areas of investigation are Alzheimer's disease and other cognitive disorders, anxiety, pain and substance abuse.

personal products; confectionaries, including chewing gums and breath mints; and shaving products, including razors and blades.

Warner-Lambert, through its Parke-Davis Group, views the hospital as the cornerstone of the healthcare delivery system. Through various exchanges with the total healthcare community, Parke-Davis has gained a deeper understanding of the forces of change at work within the healthcare industry and the challenges and opportunities that will carry over into the twenty-first century.

So that Parke-Davis will better serve hospitals' future healthcare delivery needs, it has developed a hospital advisory board, a blue-ribbon panel of industry experts assembled to increase the company's sensitivity to the evolving needs of patients and healthcare providers.

Warner-Lambert is proud to have initiated a series of executive hospital forums that gather foremost healthcare professionals and hospital executives to examine and dissect the complex issues—public policy, regulation, ethics, managed care, the aging population, reimbursement, medical technology—that confront the healthcare community.

Warner-Lambert's Parke-Davis division has been a pioneer in the prevention of coronary heart disease. It has implemented research programs in all major areas of cardiovascular risk.

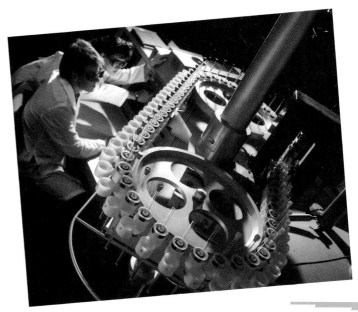

This program is accomplishing its goals; it has sparked a dynamic interchange of ideas among hospital executives, and helped set the standards for subsequent forums, including the acclaimed "National Quality of Care" forum held in Florham Park, New Jersey, in May 1992. This assembly of healthcare professionals focused on the concept of continuous quality improvement as it applies to the healthcare industry and the care of hospital patients.

Pharmaceutical discovery and development is carried out at the research center in Ann Arbor, Michigan.

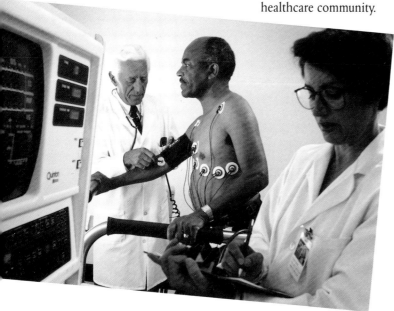

Donald F. Smith & Associates offers its sincere congratulations to the New Jersey Hospital Association for its 75 years of valuable service to healthcare facilities in the Garden State. They are very proud and grateful for the opportunity to have assisted and collaborated with the association in providing members with innovative, cost-effective insurance solutions for more than 30 years. These efforts have contributed significantly to the growth of the association.

As the leading providers of insurance programs and services to NJHA members, Donald F. Smith & Associates and Smith Insurance

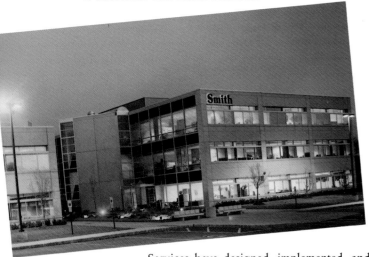

Services have designed, implemented, and administered many of the most successful insurance programs in the healthcare industry, including the first group workers' compensation and medical malpractice insurance programs for New Jersey hospitals. These programs laid the necessary foundation for the subsequent formation of the Health Care Insurance Exchange. The company also developed a unique, partially self-insured healthcare program for New Jersey hospital employees that quickly became a model followed by countless other hospitals throughout the United States.

The company's gradual expansion into the New England states, Illinois, Pennsylvania, and Virginia, came largely as a result of its work with the New Jersey Hospital Association. Using every available tool and concept to improve upon what is considered the best, they led the effort to establish Conn Med Risk Retention Company and self-insured workers' compensation trusts for hospitals in Connecticut and New Hampshire. These programs, which eliminate the vagaries of the insurance industry's pricing cycles, have collectively saved its members millions of premium dollars while providing a stable source of consistently superior protection. By concentrating on the special insurance needs of healthcare employers, they have built a reputation for efficient, results-oriented coverage and professional service that is the standard to which other brokers and consultants aspire.

With experienced, dedicated insurance professionals in healthcare insurance, retirement programs, workers' compensation, malpractice liability, errors and omissions coverage, property insurance, and all other forms of insurance protection and risk management services, Donald F. Smith & Associates and Smith Insurance Services provide full-service consulting and brokerage services to thousands of healthcare facilities, physicians, and allied health professionals across the county.

Donald F. Smith & Associates and Smith Insurance Services have offices in Lawrenceville, New Jersey; Wallingford, Connecticut; and Norfolk and Richmond, Virginia.

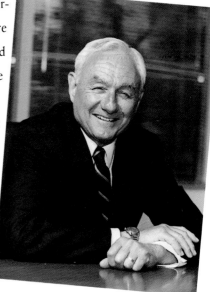

Donald F. Smith, found and chairman of the bo

For more than three decades, Giordano, Halleran & Ciesla has been a leader in the legal community. As one of the largest law firms in New Jersey, it has expanded the breadth of its legal services to meet the demands of an increasingly sophisticated client base.

The firm created its Health & Hospital Law Department 20 years ago, recognizing a critical need for legal assistance with the expanding body of complex and often restrictive laws and regulations governing New Jersey's healthcare providers. The team of specialists includes attorneys with litigation and corporate law experience, as well as former members of government regulatory agencies.

Through consultation, adjudicatory hearings, and litigation, Giordano, Halleran & Ciesla has represented the New Jersey Hospital Association for more than 15 years. The firm has been instrumental in helping to establish fundamental public policy within the regulatory framework, precedents that have helped protect the financial and professional integrity of New Jersey's healthcare providers.

A landmark case litigated successfully by the firm in 1975 helped the New Jersey Hospital Association cement a basic principle: that is, government regulators must encourage and consider comments on the broad agenda of healthcare issues, and cannot impose rules and regulations unilaterally. This principle continues to be the foundation upon which healthcare policy and hospital regulations are promulgated, affecting rate making, certificates of need, licensing, and other matters.

The firm's Health & Hospital Law team counsels its clients on a broad range of issues, utilizing its expertise in the areas of taxation, rate structuring, licensing, professional liability, managed care, medical staff issues, physician contracts, and/or corporate organizational issues.

Giordano, Halleran & Ciesla serves as general and special counsel to major medical centers, invalid carriers, home health agencies, physician groups, nursing homes, psychiatric hospitals, rehabilitative hospitals, and free-standing care centers in New Jersey.

As the range of regulations becomes more encompassing, the Health & Hospital Law team interfaces with other specialists within the firm. The issue may involve hospital waste disposal, a matter for the Environmental Law Department; a personnel matter that can be expedited by the firm's Labor & Employment Law specialists; or financing requirements handled by the firm's Public Finance group. The firm's clients are thereby assured continuity of legal counsel and representation.

Recognizing that the healthcare industry never shuts down, Giordano, Halleran & Ciesla attorneys provide 24-hour service to its clients.

Given the firm's longtime involvement in the healthcare industry and the broad scope of the firm's legal expertise, Giordano, Halleran & Ciesla is qualified to counsel its healthcare clients on the multitude of issues with which they are confronted on a daily basis.

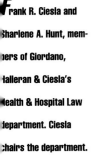

Frank R. Ciesla and Sharlene A. Hunt, members of Giordano, Halleran & Ciesla's Health & Hospital Law Department. Ciesla chairs the department.

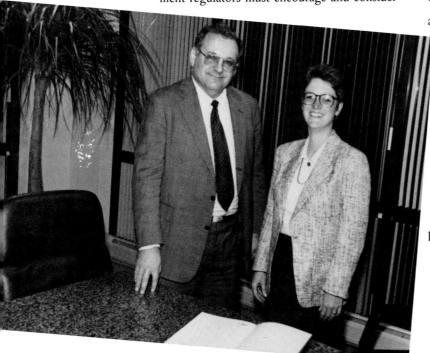

offmann-La Roche Inc., a member of the multinational family of companies headed by Roche Holding Ltd. in Basel, Switzerland, is one of the leading health-care companies in the United States. Roche has been a part of New Jersey's biomedical landscape since its U.S. corporate headquarters were established in Nutley in 1929. The company was founded on one simple principle that applies to this day: to maintain a fundamental commitment to provide the healthcare community with meaningful products and services of consistently high quality.

Quality and innovation are the building blocks upon which Roche has built an international reputation for excellence in original research and product development. Respect for this tradition has contributed to the company's strengths in basic and applied research, biotechnology, organic chemistry and biology. It also ensures that products bearing the Roche name are safe, effective, and reliable.

Roche has discovered, developed, and introduced numerous products throughout the twentieth century, including the well-known anti-anxiety medications LIBRIUM® and VALIUM®; ACCUTANE®, the breakthrough treatment for severe recalcitrant cystic acne; ROCEPHIN®, the leading injectable broad-spectrum antibiotic and most widely-used hospital pharmaceutical product; ROFERON-A®, the first recombinant human interferon product ever to enter clinical trials; and HIVID®, for use in combination therapy against AIDS.

Over the years Roche has been at the forefront of research and major developments in pharmaceuticals for the treatment of neurological problems, bacterial infections, leukemia, dermatologic disorders, and AIDS.

A major employer in New Jersey, Roche is involved in the research, development, marketing, and distribution of prescription pharmaceuticals, and is also a leader in diagnostic products and clinical testing services, vitamins and fine chemicals, and home infusion therapy services.

Recognized worldwide for excellence in biomedical science, Roche is clearly a major player in the quest for improved health and a better quality of life. Underlying its approach to drug development is the commitment to pursue innovative products that meet significant medical, patient, and societal needs. Roche also recognizes the importance of developing new medicines that are cost-effective and that can eliminate the need for surgery, shorten periods of hospitalization, reduce patients' visits to doctors, and increase patient compliance and convenience through fewer dosage regimens.

Roche is also a leader in diagnostics. Early diagnosis leading to prompt treatment can eliminate the devastating complications of advanced stages of disease and produce enormous savings in overall national medical costs. For that reason, diagnostics is one of the fastest-growing segments of the healthcare industry.

The Roche Diagnostics Group consists of three sub-

Rocephin, an injectible antibiotic developed by Roche scientists, offers a convenient once-a-day dosing regimen that has helped to make it the number one hospital pharmaceutical product on the market.

In developing important new medicines for the future, Roche employs a research and development strategy that includes b basic and applied research. A scientist in basic research studies molecular structure of cells using electron microscopy.

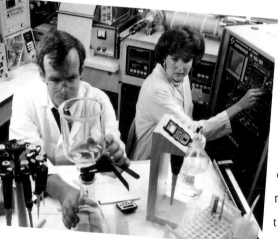

sidiaries—Roche Biomedical Laboratories, Roche Diagnostic Systems, and Roche Molecular Systems, that are leaders in the race to develop and increase the availability of new diagnostic technologies. The combined range of laboratory testing services and diagnostic reagents and instruments offered by Roche is among the most comprehensive in the healthcare industry. And, through its newest subsidiary, Roche Molecular Systems, the company is working toward the development of dramatically improved methods of disease diagnosis using a revolutionary new technology known as the polymerase chain reaction, or PCR.

Roche remains on the cutting edge of change and is committed to the pursuit of new preventative, diagnostic, and therapeutic approaches to afflictions such as cancer, AIDS, cardiovascular disease, arthritis, and Alzheimer's disease. Tackling these challenges, however, requires a laborious, lengthy, and expensive research and development process fraught with financial risk. Only about one out of every 7,000 compounds screened by scientists makes it to the marketplace. And one recent study estimated that it takes an average of 12 years and more than $230 million to develop a new medicine.

Several factors contribute to the enormous length and expense of modern drug development. Sophisticated technology today enables scientists to seek treatments and cures for chronic and degenerative diseases at the fundamental cellular level, against a backdrop of stringent, multilayered company and government regulations. This requires longer, more extensive, and more costly testing than that employed to conquer many of the acute diseases of the past.

Roche is committed to putting forth the resources and talent to continue the search for cures. Worldwide, Roche invests more than one billion dollars annually in research, providing its scientists with an intellectually stimulating environment for their work. In 1967 Roche established the first-ever corporate-funded science center devoted exclusively basic research, the Roche Institute of Molecular Biology in Nutley.

"Working Today for a Healthier Tomorrow" is more than a corporate slogan—it embodies the Roche commitment to innovative research and progressive programs that have contributed to a succession of accomplishments, discoveries, and milestones for the company and the millions of people it serves worldwide.

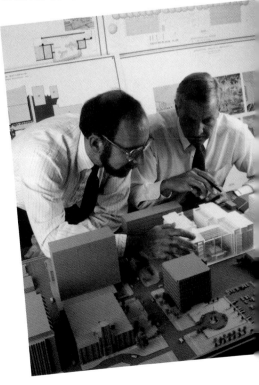

Hospitals, laboratories, and clinics generate more than 600,000 tons of biomedical waste annually in the United States. Because of its infectious nature, and the attendant problems with disposal, this waste stream of sharps, dressings, bandages, fluid packages, and other materials represents a perplexing dilemma for health care institutions. Soaring costs of disposal, liability insurance, and increased public scrutiny and government regulations must be addressed.

ABB Sanitec, a subsidiary of ABB, Inc., has developed the ABB Sanitec Microwave Disinfection System, an unobtrusive on-site disposal unit that satisfies the demand for an affordable, environmentally sound process by which hospitals can safely dispose of biomedical waste, and in so doing, both satisfy the public clamor for safety and pass rigid governmental scrutiny.

It is a cost-effective alternative to more costly methods of treatment, which involve storage and transportation of infectious wastes to off-site disposal facilities. As such, it was selected as the alternative of choice for the New Jersey Hospital Association in September 1991.

The microwave solution incorporates shredding, steam injection, and microwaves to achieve the highest levels of disinfection. There are no harmful air emissions or liquid discharges. There are no chemicals to add or dispose of. Volume is reduced by 80 percent.

The apparatus is housed in a 24-foot-long steel all-weather container. Designed to be operated by one person, the system utilizes a lift/charging system for unloading the waste material into a shredder unit via an infeed hopper assembly.

The shredded waste is injected with steam to ensure uniform absorption of heat during the treatment process. It is then pushed by a screw conveyor through a chamber where it is continually exposed to microwaves, which disinfect the waste by heating the material to a minimum 203 degrees Fahrenheit for 30 minutes. The end product, which resembles shredded bits of confetti, can then be disposed of safely in municipal landfills.

Hospitals throughout the United States, including several in New Jersey, have installed the system and are pleased with the results. Users report average processing costs of just pennies per pound, with some documenting overall savings of 80 percent over previous disposal methods.

Extensive disinfection performance studies conducted in the United States and elsewhere confirm that the processed material from the ABB Sanitec microwave units is safer than ordinary household waste.

With its proven capabilities, and with no harmful air, water, or chemical discharges to contend with, the ABB Sanitec unit meets rigid local, state, and federal environmental standards; as such, it can be shipped, installed, and operating in short order.

ABB Sanitec provides complete on-site training for operating and maintenance personnel, offering full guarantees and its own staff of engineers and technicians to assure that each unit operates at the optimum.

Cooper Hospital in Camden was one of the first hospitals in New Jersey to employ ABB Sanitec Microwave Disinfection technology to treat its red bag waste.

The ABB Sanitec system employs advanced shredding technology with conventional microwave energy to render waste both thoroughly unrecognizable and completely disinfected.

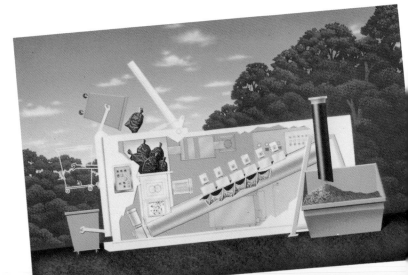

Since 1983 the Hyatt Regency Princeton has been a noted landmark along the Route 1 corridor in West Windsor. Located in Carnegie Center, it is midway between New York and Philadelphia and conveniently nestled in an area rich in historical significance and corporate tenants.

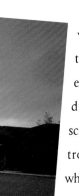

The beautifully landscaped front drive of the Hyatt Regency Princeton.

This five-story luxury hotel has 348 beautifully appointed sleeping rooms; 10 suites, including an exquisite Presidential Suite; a 10,000-square-foot ballroom; 12,000 square feet of additional meeting space; a restaurant connected to a wine bar; a multilevel cocktail lounge; and nightly entertainment in the comedy club. The lushly landscaped atrium lobby creates a tropical haven for patrons who come to "get away from it all" for lunch, dinner, or cocktails, or to discuss business in a comfortable setting. The property is owned and operated by Hyatt Hotels Corporation of Chicago.

The hotel's tasteful landscaping and exterior architecture reflect Carnegie Center's overall high standards and design. Inside, guests are treated to a sky-lighted atrium that is split by a stairway and waterfall, along which is the multilevel Water's Edge cocktail lounge. At the bottom of the staircase is the Crystal Garden Cafe, which now has a fresh and colorful look with an Art Nouveau influence in decor, and affordable, innovative new menu items for breakfast, lunch, and dinner. Sunday Brunch in the Crystal Garden features traditional breakfast treats and creative and delicious lunch selections, served in the atrium lobby.

Recessed in the Main Lobby and connected to the Crystal Garden Cafe, the By The Glass wine bar is an innovative concept offering an impressive collection of French and California wines and Champagnes by the glass. Lively entertainment can be found nightly at the legendary comedy club, Catch A Rising Star.

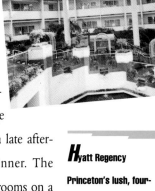

On the second floor overlooking the atrium, the Regency Club lounge is a relaxing spot for morning coffee, a late afternoon snack, or a cocktail before dinner. The Regency Club, consisting of upgraded rooms on a private floor, offers upgraded amenities and use of the Regency Club lounge and concierge services.

Hyatt Regency Princeton's lush, four-story atrium and The Water's Edge Lounge.

The Hyatt Regency Princeton hosts many prestigious annual charity events and has historically been a leader in the area's fund-raising efforts, supporting such worthy pursuits as the Eden Institute for Autism, American Cancer Society, United Way, March of Dimes, and the New Jersey Hospital Association.

Central New Jersey and nearby Pennsylvania are rich with historical landmarks, monuments, and architecture. Guests can visit landmarks both in Princeton and in New Hope, in scenic Bucks County, Pennsylvania. With the Princeton Junction railroad station just a mile from the hotel, Hyatt Regency Princeton's prime location affords guests easy access to Philadelphia and New York via Amtrak. The famed Jersey shore and Atlantic City are also within driving distance, as well as Six Flags Great Adventure in Jackson, New Jersey, and Sesame Place in nearby Langhorne, Pennsylvania.

This lovely hotel in the cultural center of the Garden State is the perfect place to experience the "Hyatt Touch."

Located midway between New York and Philadelphia along the prestigious Route 1 corridor, the Princeton Marriott is the focal point of Princeton Forrestal Village, a bustling center of leisure, commerce, and business that is patterned after a turn-of-the-century village in the shadows of the Ivy League towers on the Princeton University campus.

Fountains, colorful awnings, brick walkways, a pedestrian plaza, flower beds, and extensive landscaping offer a pleasant respite from the demands and rigors of travel and the business day. Travelers can enjoy an evening at either of the hotel's two restaurants, and a bevy of upscale outlet stores recently opened in the village adds to the eclectic appeal of the many diversions.

Here you'll find quality, service, and friendly, courteous staff, eager to help. It's a modern, sophisticated meeting place with an old-fashioned look, an environment offering the best in business and pleasure.

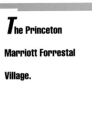

The Princeton Marriott Forrestal Village.

Its location is ideally suited to Central New Jersey's high concentration of *Fortune* 500 corporate offices and research facilities, as well as the state capital in nearby Trenton, and the outstanding academic neighbors, Princeton University and Rutgers, the state university in New Brunswick.

Its well-appointed facilities provide a workplace away from the office, and a home away from home, with the subtle emphasis on convenience, efficiency, and comfort. It is geared to handle the rigid demands of multinational corporations, as well as those of the overnight business traveler. It is also the perfect destination for a romantic weekend getaway or a relaxing family vacation.

Hospitality at the Princeton Marriott comes wrapped in all shapes and sizes, from its 9,880-square-foot Forrestal Ballroom to the intimacy of its 292 well-appointed guest rooms and suites. Each room is equipped with color television, cable service, and in-room pay movies.

There are also an indoor/outdoor pool and well-equipped health club for after-meeting fitness and family fun. And there are a jogging path and softball fields for corporate fun and games.

Inside, beyond the well-appointed lobby, is the Concierge Level, which includes a private lounge for complimentary Continental breakfasts and afternoon hors d'oeuvres. Located here are four suites perfectly appointed for small executive sessions or VIP dinners.

There's the Village Green for casual dining; and for exotic Japanese Teppanyaki dining, there's Mikado's. The Lobby Lounge sets a quiet tone for discussing the day's business, while Boomerang's features a sophisticated sound system, video, and contemporary decor to help with unwinding at the end of a long, hard day. It's a popular after-work gathering place for the area's professionals.

Grand enough to accommodate 1,600 for a reception, the Forrestal Ballroom can be divided into eight soundproof sections, ideal for smaller corporate gatherings. Flexibility is the key, with hospitality suites, seven meet-

Forrestal Village offers a pleasing combination of fountains, colorful awnings, brick walkways, a pedestrian plaza, flower beds, and extensive landscaping.

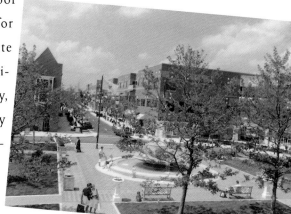

ing rooms, and registration and reception areas available throughout the property.

Marriott-style service begins with a single call to an Executive Meeting Manager, adept at handling details big and small: guest accommodations, meeting room setups, audiovisual support, creative theme parties, teleconferencing, limousine service, airport connections, fresh flowers, even a crisply pressed shirt.

The Princeton Marriott's experienced staff is trained to anticipate all needs at this world-class facility, and is backed up by an efficient infrastructure and Marriott's time honored traditions of first-class service.

From its modest beginnings in 1927 as a nine-seat root beer stand in Washington, D.C., the Marriott Corporation has grown into the world's leading hospitality company, with lodging and other related companies operating in all 50 states and 17 countries.

Widely recognized as one of the best-managed companies in the United States, it has nearly 230,000 employees, making Marriott one of the 10 largest employers in the United States. Marriott is the world's largest operator of hotel rooms and offers a diversified range of short- and long-term lodging products, totaling 539 hotels with more than 134,000 rooms.

Marriott Hotels and Resorts are full-service hotels, resorts, and suites serving guests in the luxury and quality segment of the market, usually located in downtown, suburban, and airport sites.

Courtyard by Marriott is designed for the business traveler, and is considered the company's moderate hotel product.

Residence Inn is the company's extended-stay facility, designed for guests relocating to a new city, working on a temporary long-term assignment, or attending a seminar or training assignment. Individual units are designed to provide home-like comforts, including fully equipped kitchens.

Marriott's Fairfield Inns, first opened in 1987, offer economy-priced lodging, and are already a leader in this segment of the market.

Marriott Ownership Resorts offer time-sharing facilities for families, with projects in Hilton Head, South Carolina; Palm Springs, California; and Orlando, Florida. Plans call for several more to be built in the 1990s, including Vail, Colorado; and Puerto Vallarta, Mexico.

Marriott also offers a full range of contract food service and management, serving nearly 2,300 clients. Food service operations include employee cafeterias, executive dining facilities, stadiums, and sports arenas. Host International operates cafeterias, snack bars, restaurants, gift shops, and newsstands at U.S. and foreign airport terminals, while Marriott Travel Plazas operates more than 100 restaurants, gift shops, and related facilities on 14 major highway systems in the United States.

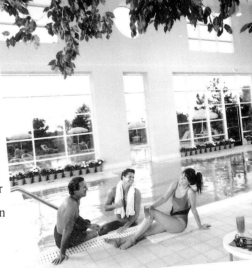

E mergency Medical Associates (EMA) of New Jersey is a professional group of physicians that specializes in emergency medical care, a unique group practice that provides emergency department staffing and management for nearly a dozen hospitals in New Jersey.

Since its founding in 1976, EMA has responded to the ever-changing dynamics of the healthcare delivery system by anticipating long-term needs of the partnership, its clients, and the hundreds of thousands of patients its doctors treat annually.

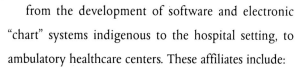

This natural progression has seen several EMA affiliates evolve, each with its own specialty, generating a variety of services, from the development of software and electronic "chart" systems indigenous to the hospital setting, to ambulatory healthcare centers. These affiliates include:

• Emergency Medical Offices, which staffs and manages ambulatory-care centers in three New Jersey locations: Middletown, Berkeley Heights, and Riverdale.

• Emergency Medical Billing, which offers assistance to both hospitals and physician groups in the complex area of direct patient billing, emergency medicine billing, and reimbursement. Since 1980 EMB has consulted on a number of billing systems for individual hospitals, and has provided full-service turnkey operations for others. It currently services 25 hospitals in New Jersey, New York, and Pennsylvania.

• Emergency Medical Associates Research Foundation, which cooperates with the Emergency Medicine Residency program and the other EMA affiliates in

order to assist, promote, and coordinate emergency medicine seminars and research.

• Emergency Medical Consultants, which can provide house physicians for hospitals requiring such services, on temporary or long-term basis.

Unlike other emergency medical practices that employ physicians, the majority of EMA is wholly owned by its member physicians. All newly employed physicians are eligible to enter into shareholder status following the completion of their second year of full-time employment, and continue to full partnership with additional shares acquisition. This process is used to ensure the continued, dedicated involvement of EMA's physicians.

EMA utilizes the services of 61 physicians, whose average age is 41, with an average length of service with EMA of seven years. EMA emphasizes the contracting of physicians who have obtained, or will obtain, proper certification from the American Board of Emergency Medicine. Currently 82 percent of EMA physicians are ABEM certified; the remainder are ABEM residency prepared or practice prepared.

EMA has steered a course of calculated, measured growth, avoiding the temptation to expand too quickly. "The quality of the group is paramount. It drives what we do," explains EMA President Peter L. Sawchuk, M.D. "We have tried not to grow so fast that we can't attract the kind of physicians we're looking for."

All prospective emergency medical department physicians are presented to the client hospital's medical staff committee for approval. Once accepted, the physician becomes a member of the

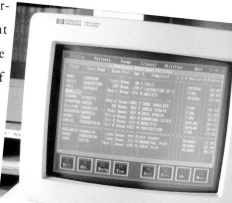

medical staff and must submit to all standards and by-laws in effect at that hospital. EMA physicians have no admitting privileges and are not permitted any outside medical interests that could conflict with their career in emergency medicine.

EMA physicians staff and manage the emergency departments at Mountainside Hospital, EMA's first client; Bayshore Community Hospital; Hackensack Medical Center; Morristown Memorial Hospital; Muhlenberg Regional Medical Center; Robert Wood Johnson University Hospital; Saint Barnabas Medical Center; St Clares* Riverside Medical Center; and

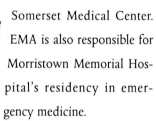

Somerset Medical Center. EMA is also responsible for Morristown Memorial Hospital's residency in emergency medicine.

EMA recognizes the significant role its physicians play in the positive interaction of a hospital within the New Jersey Emergency Medical System. In all its hospitals, EMA works closely with regional ambulance and rescue squads through participation in regularly scheduled squad meetings, captain's meetings, educational programs, and daily interaction in the emergency department when the volunteers arrive with a patient in need of immediate care.

EMA has continually demonstrated its ability to provide medical management and control, supervision, training, communications, operations reviews, evaluations, and quality of Mobile Intensive Care Units based at its client hospitals.

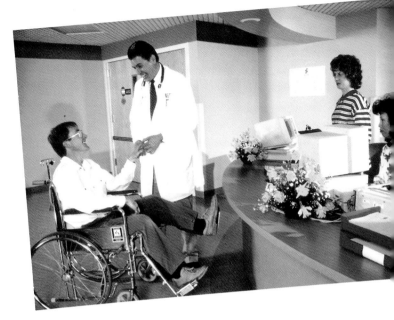

EMA physicians are expected to take an active role in assuring the efficient operation of the emergency department. EMA encourages their involvement in such areas as:

• Supervision of quality improvement activities;

• Recommendations regarding equipment acquisition and staffing;

• Staff development activities, including sanctioned in-service education programs;

• Leadership and coordination in the development of policies and protocols;

• Community involvement with local ambulance and rescue squads to help enhance pre- hospital care;

• Evaluation and response to all patient inquiries regarding the services of the emergency department.

EMA and its affiliates have positioned themselves to respond to the ever-changing dynamics and increasing demands placed on the emergency medicine departments of their hospitals well into the 21st century. EMA, together with its affiliates, will continue its dedication to the quality clinical practice of emergency medicine.

The following individuals, companies, and organizations have made a valuable commitment to the quality of this publication. The publisher and the New Jersey Hospital Association gratefully acknowledge their participation in *The New Jersey Hospital Association 75th Anniversary* CELEBRATING INNOVATIVE LEADERSHIP IN HEALTHCARE.

PARTNERS IN PROGRESS

ABB Sanitec, Inc., *132*
Barre National, *110*
Emergency Medical Associates, *136*
Emergency Physician Associates, *102*
GHR Consulting Services, *114*
Giordano, Halleran & Ciesla, *129*
Health Care Insurance Company, *101*
Hoescht-Roussel Pharmaceuticals, *120*
Hoffmann-La Roche, *130*
Hyatt Regency Princeton, *133*
Immuno-U.S., Inc., *108*
Johnson & Johnson, *104*
Kabi Pharmacia, Inc., *118*
National Medical Rental Leasing & Sales, Inc., *113*
National Westminster Bank, *112*
New Jersey Hospital Association, *100*
Office Business Systems, *119*
Princeton Marriott Forrestal Village, *134*
Schein Pharmaceutical, Inc., *111*
Schering-Plough, *122*
ServiceMaster Management Services, *107*
Donald F. Smith & Associates, *128*
SmithKline Beecham Pharmaceuticals, *116*
UMDNJ, *124*
Warner-Lambert Co., *126*

SPECIAL CONTRIBUTOR

CONGRATULATIONS
and best wishes on
75 successful years.

Multiplan Inc.
Donald Rubin,
President

PATRONS

Abbott Laboratories
A. E. Litho Group/Riverside Graphics
Blickman Health Industries, Inc.
BLM Group
Cetus Corporation
Connaught Laboratories
E. Fougera & Company
Geneva Marsam
Goldline Laboratories, Inc.
Hannoch Weisman
McGaw, Inc.
National Hospital Specialties
Nihon Kohden America, Inc.
Purdue-Frederick Company
Sherwood Medical Company
Smith-Nephew United Inc.
UDL Laboratories, Inc.
United Jersey Bank
Xactdose, Inc.

HOSPITAL AND INSTITUTIONAL MEMBERS*

A **Ancora Psychiatric Hospital** *(Founded 1955)* 202 Spring Garden Road, Ancora, NJ 08037-9699, (609) 561-1700, William Camarota, Chief Executive Officer

Atlantic City Medical Center *(Founded 1897)* 1925 Pacific Avenue, Atlantic City, NJ 08401, (609) 344-4081, George F. Lynn, President

    Mainland Division of Atlantic City Medical Center *(Founded 1975)* Jim Leeds Road, Pomona, NJ 08240, (609) 652-1000

B **Barnert Hospital** *(Founded 1908)* 680 Broadway, Paterson, NJ 07514, (201) 977-6600, Fred L. Lang, President and CEO

Bayonne Hospital *(Founded 1888)* 29 East 29th Street, Bayonne, NJ 07002, (201) 858-5000, Michael R. D'Agnes, President and CEO

Bayshore Community Hospital *(Founded 1972)* 727 North Beers Street, Holmdel, NJ 07733, (908) 739-5900, Thomas Goldman, President

Bergen Pines County Hospital *(Founded 1914)* 230 East Ridgewood Avenue, Paramus, NJ 07652, (201) 967-4000, Edward M. Lewis, Chief Executive Officer

Beth Israel Hospital *(Founded 1926)* 70 Parker Avenue, Passaic, NJ 07055, (201) 365-5000, Jeffrey Moll, President and CEO

Betty Bacharach Rehabilitation Hospital *(Founded 1924)* Jim Leeds Road, Pomona, NJ 08240, (609) 652-7000, Richard J. Kathrins, Administrator

Burdette Tomlin Memorial Hospital *(Founded 1950)* Stone Harbor Boulevard, Cape May Court House, NJ 08210, (609) 463-2000, Thomas L. Scott, FACHE, President and CEO

Buttonwood Hospital of Burlington County *(Founded 1900)* Evergreen Park/Buttonwood Hall, Route 530, Pemberton-Browns Mills Road, New Lisbon, NJ 08064, (609) 726-7000, Donald Hillegas, Hospital Superintendent

C **Camden County Health Services Center** *(Founded 1916)* Executive Offices, Collier Drive, Blackwood, NJ 08012, (609) 757-8000, Anthony Peters, Chief Executive Officer

Carrier Foundation *(Founded 1900)* County Route 601, P.O. Box 147, Belle Mead, NJ 08502, (908) 281-1000, Stanley J. Birch, Jr., C.P.A., President and CEO

Cathedral Healthcare System, Inc. One Gateway Center, Suite 2600, Newark, NJ 07102-5311, (201) 642-5100, Sister Margaret J. Straney, R.S.M., President and CEO

    Cathedral Health Services, Inc.:

    Saint James Hospital Division *(Founded 1900)* 155 Jefferson Street, Newark, NJ 07105, (201) 589-1300

    Saint Mary's Ambulatory Care Hospital Division *(Founded 1989)* 135 South Center Street, Orange, NJ 07050, (201) 266-3000

    Saint Michael's Medical Center Division *(Founded 1867)* 268 Dr. Martin Luther King Jr. Boulevard, Newark, NJ 07102, (201) 877-5000

Catholic Community Services *(Founded 1928)* Mount Carmel Guild, 17 Mulberry Street, Newark, NJ 07102, (201) 596-4100, Msgr. Nicholas DiMarzio, Ph.D., Executive Director

CentraState Healthcare System, 901 West Main Street, Freehold, NJ 07728-2549, (908) 431-2000, Thomas H. Litz, FACHE, President and CEO

    CentraState Medical Center *(Founded 1971)* 901 West Main Street, Freehold, NJ 07728-2549, (908) 431-2000

Children's Specialized Hospital *(Founded 1891)* 150 New Providence Road, Mountainside, NJ 07092-2590, (908) 233-3720, Richard B. Ahlfeld, President

Chilton Memorial Hospital *(Founded 1947)* 97 West Parkway, Pompton Plains, NJ 07444, (201) 831-5000, James J. Doyle, Jr., President and CEO

Christ Hospital *(Founded 1874)* 176 Palisade Avenue, Jersey City, NJ 07306, (201) 795-8200, Lloyd R. Currier, President

Christian Health Care Center *(Founded 1911)* 301 Sicomac Avenue, Wyckoff, NJ 07481, (201) 848-5200, Robert Van Dyk, President and CEO

    Heritage Manor East and West Nursing Home *(Founded 1954)* 301 Sicomac Avenue, Wyckoff, NJ 07481; (201) 848-5200, Denise B. Ratcliffe, Executive Vice President and Administrator

    Ramapo Ridge Psychiatric Hospital *(Founded 1911)* 301 Sicomac Avenue, Wyckoff, NJ 07481, (201) 848-5200, Joan P. Craper, Administrator and Executive Vice President

Clara Maass Medical Center *(Founded 1868)* One Franklin Avenue, Belleville, NJ 07109, (201) 450-2000, Robert S. Curtis, President and CEO

Columbus Hospital *(Founded 1934)* 495 North 13th Street, Newark, NJ 07107, (201) 268-1400, John G. Magliaro, Administrator

Community Medical Center *(Founded 1961)* 99 Highway 37 West, Toms River, NJ 08755, (908) 240-8000, Mark D. Pilla, President and CEO

Community Mental Health Center at Piscataway–UMDNJ *(Founded 1972)* 671 Hoes Lane, P.O. Box 1392, Piscataway, NJ 08855-1392, (908) 463-4338, Gary W. Lamson, Vice President and CEO for Mental Health Services

Cooper Hospital/University Medical Center *(Founded 1866)* One Cooper Plaza, Camden, NJ 08103, (609) 342-2000, Kevin G. Halpern, President and CEO

D **Daughters of Miriam Center for the Aged** *(Founded 1921)* 155 Hazel Street, Clifton, NJ 07015, (201) 772-3700, Harvey Adelsberg, Executive Vice President

Deborah Heart and Lung Center *(Founded 1922)* Trenton Road, Browns Mills, NJ 08015, (609) 893-6611, John R. Ernst, Executive Director

Dover General Hospital and Medical Center *(Founded 1908)* Jardine Street, Dover, NJ 07801, (201) 989-3000, Wayne C. Schiffner, President

E **East Orange General Hospital** *(Founded 1903)* 300 Central Avenue, East Orange, NJ 07019, (201) 672-8400, Laurence M. Merlis, President and CEO

Elizabeth General Medical Center *(Founded 1879)* 925 East Jersey Street, Elizabeth, NJ 07201, (908) 289-8600, David A. Fletcher, President and CEO

Elmer Community Hospital *(Founded 1950)* West Front Street, P.O. Box 1090, Elmer, NJ 08318, (609) 358-2341, John H. Wisda, Administrator

Englewood Hospital *(Founded 1888)* 350 Engle Street, Englewood, NJ 07631, (201) 894-3000, Daniel A. Kane, Dr.P.H., President and CEO

Essex County Hospital Center *(Founded 1872)* 125 Fairview Avenue, Cedar Grove, NJ 07009, (201) 228-8000, Michael P. Duffy, Director, Department of Health and Rehabilitation

The Estaugh *(Founded 1914)* Medford Leas, Route 70, Medford, NJ 08055, (609) 654-3000, Lois Forrest, Executive Director

F **Fair Oaks Hospital** *(Founded 1902)* 19 Prospect Street, Summit, NJ 07901, (908) 522-7000, Richard G. Jensen, Chief Executive Officer

Francis E. Parker Memorial Home *(Founded 1907)* Easton Avenue at Landing Lane, New Brunswick, NJ 08901, (908) 545-3110, Robert M. Piegari, President

Franciscan Health System of New Jersey, Inc. Corporate Office, One McWilliams Place, Jersey City, NJ 07302, (201) 714-8900, Ulrich J. Rosa, President and CEO

as of 12/31/92

St. Francis Hospital *(Founded 1864)* 25 McWilliams Place, Jersey City, NJ 07302, (201) 714-8900

St. Mary Hospital *(Founded 1863)* 308 Willow Avenue, Hoboken, NJ 07030, (201) 714-8900

G

Garden State Rehabilitation Hospital *(Founded 1974)* 14 Hospital Drive, Toms River, NJ 08755, (908) 244-3100, David M. Coluzzi, CEO and Administrator

The General Hospital Center at Passaic *(Founded 1892)* 350 Boulevard, Passaic, NJ 07055, (201) 365-4300, Daniel L. Marcantuono, President and CEO

Graduate Health System Inc. Corporate Office, 22nd & Chestnut streets, Philadelphia, PA 19103, (215) 448-1500, Robert E. Mathews, President and COO

Rancocas Hospital *(Founded 1961)* Sunset Road, Willingboro, NJ 08046, (609) 835-2900, Garry L. Scheib, President

Zurbrugg Hospital *(Founded 1915)* Hospital Plaza, Riverside, NJ 08075, (609) 461-6700, Bernadette M. Mangan, President

Green Hill *(Founded 1867)* 103 Pleasant Valley Way, West Orange, NJ 07052, (201) 731-2300, Marie E. Powell, Ph.D., Executive Director

Greenville Hospital *(Founded 1912)* 1825 Kennedy Boulevard, Jersey City, NJ 07305, (201) 547-6100, Jonathan M. Metsch, Dr.P.H., President and CEO

Greystone Park Psychiatric Hospital *(Founded 1876)* Greystone Park, NJ 07950 , (201) 538-1800, Colonel George A. Waters, Jr., CEO

Grotta Center for Senior Care *(Founded 1922)* 20 Summit Street, West Orange, NJ 07052, (201) 736-2000, Harriet Gaidemak, R.N., Ph.D., L.N.H.A., Executive Director

H

Hackensack Medical Center *(Founded 1888)* 30 Prospect Avenue, Hackensack, NJ 07601, (201) 996-2000, John P. Ferguson, FACHE, President and CEO

Hasbrouck Heights Facility, 214 Terrace Avenue, Hasbrouck Heights, NJ 07604, (201) 288-0800

Hackettstown Community Hospital *(Founded 1973)* 651 Willow Grove Street, Hackettstown, NJ 07840-1792, (908) 852-5100, Gene C. Milton, President and CEO

Hamilton Hospital *(Founded 1936)* Hamilton Center for Health, 1881 White-Horse Hamilton Square Road, Hamilton, NJ 08690, (609) 586-7900, W. Michael Bryant, C.P.A., M.B.A., President and CEO

Hampton Hospital *(Founded 1986)* P.O. Box 7000, Rancocas Road, Rancocas, NJ 08073, (609) 267-7000, John Watkins, CEO and Administrator

Helene Fuld Medical Center *(Founded 1887)* 750 Brunswick Avenue, Trenton, NJ 08638, (609) 394-6000, William K. Hogan, President and CEO

Holy Name Hospital *(Founded 1925)* 718 Teaneck Road, Teaneck, NJ 07666, (201) 833-3000, Sister Patricia Lynch, CSJP, President and CEO

The Hospital Center at Orange *(Founded 1873)* 188 South Essex Avenue, Orange, NJ 07051, (201) 266-2000, Arthur T. Dunn, President

Hunterdon Medical Center *(Founded 1954)* Route 31, Flemington, NJ 08822, (908) 788-6100, Robert P. Wise, President and CEO

I

Irvington General Hospital *(Founded 1924)* 832 Chancellor Avenue, Irvington, NJ 07111, (201) 399-6000, Frank L. Muddle, President and CEO

Jersey City Medical Center *(Founded 1868)* 50 Baldwin Avenue, Jersey City, NJ 07304, (201) 915-2000, Jonathan M. Metsch, Dr.P.H., President and CEO

J

Jersey Shore Medical Center *(Founded 1904)* 1945 Route 33, Neptune, NJ 07754, (908) 775-5500, John K. Lloyd, President

Jewish Home and Rehabilitation Center *(Founded 1915)* 198 Stevens Avenue, Jersey City, NJ 07305, (201) 451-9000, Charles P. Berkowitz, Executive Vice President

Jewish Home and Rehabilitation Center *(Founded 1970)* 685 Westwood Avenue, River Vale, NJ 07675, (201) 666-2370, Ellen Ress, Administrator

JFK Health Systems Inc. Corporate Offices, Mediplex Suite 400, 98 James Street, Edison, NJ 08820-3998, (908) 632-1500, John P. McGee, President and CEO

John F. Kennedy Medical Center *(Founded 1967)* 65 James Street, Edison, NJ 08817, (908) 321-7000

JFK Johnson Rehabilitation Institute *(Founded 1974)* 65 James Street, Edison, NJ 08817, (908) 321-7050, Scott Gebhard, Administrator

K

Kennedy Memorial Hospitals–University Medical Center, Corporate Office, 500 Marlboro Avenue, P.O. Box 5087, Cherry Hill, NJ 08034-5087, (609) 661-5100, Richard E. Murray, President and CEO

Cherry Hill Division *(Founded 1960)* 2201 Chapel Avenue, P.O. Box 5009, Cherry Hill, NJ 08002-2048, (609) 488-6500

Stratford Division *(Founded 1965)* 18 East Laurel Road, Stratford, NJ 08084, (609) 346-6000

Washington Township Division *(Founded 1972)* Hurffville-Cross Keys Road, Turnersville, NJ 08012, (609) 582-2500

Kessler Institute for Rehabilitation *(Founded 1949)* Corporate Office, 1199 Pleasant Valley Way, West Orange, NJ 07052, (201) 731-3600, Kenneth W. Aitchison, President

Kessler Institute for Rehabilitation–Kessler East *(Founded 1982)* Central Avenue and the Parkway, East Orange, NJ 07018, (201) 731-3600

Kessler Institute for Rehabilitation–Kessler North *(Founded 1986)* 300 Market Street, Saddle Brook, NJ 07662, (201) 587-8500

Kessler Institute for Rehabilitation–Kessler West *(Founded 1948)* 1199 Pleasant Valley Way, West Orange, NJ 07052, (201) 731-3600

M

Marlboro Psychiatric Hospital *(Founded 1930)* Station A, Marlboro, NJ 07746, (908) 946-8100, Michael Ross, Ph.D., Chief Executive Officer

The Matheny School *(Founded 1946)* Main Street, Peapack, NJ 07977, (908) 234-0011, Robert Schonhorn, President

Meadowlands Hospital Medical Center *(Founded 1944)* Meadowland Parkway, Secaucus, NJ 07096-1580, (201) 392-3100, Helen M. Kennedy, President and CEO

Meadow View Nursing and Convalescent Center *(Founded 1988)* 1328 S. Black Horse Pike, Williamstown, NJ 08094, (609) 875-0100, Peter J. Burke, Jr., President

The Medical Center at Princeton *(Founded 1919)* 253 Witherspoon Street, Princeton, NJ 08540-3213, (609) 497-4000, Dennis W. Doody, President and CEO

The Medical Center of Ocean County, Inc. 2121 Edgewater Place, Point Pleasant, NJ 08742-2290, (908) 892-1100, John T. Gribbon, President

Brick Hospital Division *(Founded 1983)* 425 Jack Martin Boulevard, Bricktown, NJ 08723, (908) 840-2200

Point Pleasant Hospital Division *(Founded 1929)* 2121 Edgewater Place, Point Pleasant, NJ 08742-2290, (908) 892-1100

Mediplex Rehab–Camden *(Founded 1984)* Two Cooper Plaza, Camden, NJ 08103, (609) 342-7600, David W. Ellis, Ph.D., CEO

Memorial Health Alliance Inc. Corporate Office, 175 Madison Avenue, Mount Holly, NJ 08060, (609) 261-7011, Chester B. Kaletkowski, President and CEO

Memorial Hospital of Burlington County *(Founded 1880)* 175 Madison Avenue, Mount Holly, NJ 08060, (609) 267-0700

The Memorial Hospital of Salem County, Inc. *(Founded 1919)* Salem-Woodstown Road, Salem, NJ 08079, (609) 935-1000, Jos. Michael Galvin, Jr., FACHE, President and CEO

The Mercer Medical Center *(Founded 1895)* 446 Bellevue Avenue, Trenton, NJ 08607, (609) 394-4000, Charles E. Baer, President

Monmouth Medical Center *(Founded 1887)* 300 Second Avenue, Long Branch, NJ 07740, (908) 222-5200, Christopher M. Dadlez, FACHE, President and CEO

Montclair Community Hospital *(Founded 1923)* 120 Harrison Avenue, Montclair, NJ 07042, (201) 744-7300, Emilie M. Murphy, Director

Morristown Memorial Hospital *(Founded 1892)* 100 Madison Avenue, P.O. Box 1956, Morristown, NJ 07962-1956, (201) 971-5000, Richard P. Oths, President and CEO

>   **Mt. Kemble Division of Morristown Memorial Hospital** *(Founded circa 1890)* (Formerly All Souls Hospital) 95 Mt. Kemble Avenue, P.O. Box 1978, Morristown, NJ 07962-1978, (201) 971-4400

The Mountainside Hospital *(Founded 1891)* Bay & Highland Avenues, Montclair, NJ 07042, (201) 429-6000, Bernard G. Koval, President and CEO

Muhlenberg Regional Medical Center *(Founded 1877)* Park Avenue & Randolph Road, P.O. Box 1272, Plainfield, NJ 07061, (908) 668-2000, John R. Kopicki, President and CEO

N **Newark Beth Israel Medical Center** *(Founded 1901)* 201 Lyons Avenue, Newark, NJ 07112, (201) 926-7000, Lester M. Bornstein, President

Newcomb Medical Center *(Founded 1908)* 65 South State Street, Vineland, NJ 08360, (609) 691-9000, Joseph A. Ierardi, President and CEO

Newton Memorial Hospital *(Founded 1932)* 175 High Street, Newton, NJ 07860, (201) 383-2121, Dennis H. Collette, President and CEO

O **Our Lady of Lourdes Medical Center** *(Founded 1950)* 1600 Haddon Avenue, Camden, NJ 08103, (609) 757-3500, Alexander J. Hatala, Chief Executive Officer

Overlook Hospital *(Founded 1906)* 99 Beauvoir Avenue at 41 Sylvan Road, Summit, NJ 07901-0220, (908) 522-2000, Michael J. Sniffen, President and CEO

P **Palisades General Hospital** *(Founded 1901)* 7600 River Road, North Bergen, NJ 07047, (201) 854-5000, William R. Friedman, President and CEO

Pascack Valley Hospital (See **Well Care Group, Inc.**)

Patterson Army Community Hospital *(Founded 1917)* Fort Monmouth, NJ 07703-5000, (908) 532-1266, LTC Martin J. Fisher, Deputy Commander for Administration

Presbyterian Homes of New Jersey Foundation and Affiliates *(Founded 1916)* Corporate Office, P.O. Box 2184, 103 Carnegie Center, Suite 300, Princeton, NJ 08543, (609) 987-8900, Thomas F. LePrevost, President and CEO

R **Rahway Hospital** *(Founded 1916)* 865 Stone Street, Rahway, NJ 07065, (908) 381-4200, John L. Yoder, President

Ramapo Ridge Psychiatric Hospital (See **Christian Health Care Center**)

Rancocas Valley Hospital (See **Graduate Health System, Inc.**)

Raritan Bay Medical Center *(Founded 1902)* 530 New Brunswick Avenue, Perth Amboy, NJ 08861, (908) 442-3700, Keith H. McLaughlin, President and CEO

>   **Old Bridge Division** *(Founded 1979)* One Hospital Plaza, Old Bridge, NJ 08857, (908) 360-1000
>   **Perth Amboy Division** *(Founded 1888)* 530 New Brunswick Avenue, Perth Amboy, NJ 08861, (908) 442-3700

Riverview Medical Center *(Founded 1922)* One Riverview Plaza, Red Bank, NJ 07701, (908) 741-2700, John K. Pawlowski, President and CEO

Robert Wood Johnson University Hospital *(Founded 1884)* One Robert Wood Johnson Place, New Brunswick, NJ 08901, (908) 828-3000, Harvey A. Holzberg, President and CEO

Roosevelt Hospital *(Founded 1936)* P.O. Box 151, Metuchen, NJ 08840, (908) 321-6800, Thomas J. Romeo, Superintendent and CEO

Runnells Specialized Hospital *(Founded 1912)* 40 Watchung Way, Berkeley Heights, NJ 07922, (908) 771-5700, Joseph W. Sharp, Hospital Administrator

S **Saint Barnabas Medical Center** *(Founded 1865)* 94 Old Short Hills Road, Livingston, NJ 07039, (201) 533-5000, Ronald J. Del Mauro, President and CEO

Saint James Hospital (See **Cathedral Healthcare System, Inc.**)

Saint Mary's Hospital (Orange) (See **Cathedral Healthcare System, Inc.**)

Saint Michael's Medical Center (See **Cathedral Healthcare System, Inc.**)

St Clares* Riverside Medical Center *(Founded 1953)* Corporate Office, Pocono Road, Denville, NJ 07834, (201) 625-6000, Joseph A. Trunfio, Ph.D., President

>   **Boonton Division** Powerville Road, Boonton, NJ 07005, (201) 334-5000
>   **Denville Division** *(Founded 1953)* Pocono Road, Denville, NJ 07834, (201) 625-6000

St. Elizabeth Hospital *(Founded 1905)* 225 Williamson Street, Elizabeth, NJ 07207, (908) 527-5000, Sister Elizabeth Ann Maloney, President and CEO

St. Francis Hospital (Jersey City) (See **Franciscan Health System of New Jersey, Inc.**)

St. Francis Medical Center *(Founded 1874)* 601 Hamilton Avenue, Trenton, NJ 08629-1986, (609) 599-5000, Patrick F. Roche, President

St. Joseph's Hospital and Medical Center *(Founded 1867)* 703 Main Street, Paterson, NJ 07503, (201) 977-2000, Sister Jane Frances Brady, President

St. Lawrence Rehabilitation Center *(Founded 1909)* 2381 Lawrenceville Road, Lawrenceville, NJ 08648, (609) 896-9500, Charles L. Brennan, Chief Executive Officer

St. Mary Hospital (Hoboken) (See **Franciscan Health System of New Jersey, Inc.**)

St. Mary's Hospital Passaic *(Founded 1895)* 211 Pennington Avenue, Passaic, NJ 07055, (201) 470-3000, Hugh Quigley, President and CEO

St. Peter's Medical Center *(Founded 1907)* 254 Easton Avenue, P.O. Box 591, New Brunswick, NJ 08903, (908) 745-8600, John Matuska, President and CEO

Seabrook House, Inc. *(Founded 1974)* P.O. Box 5055, Polk Lane, Seabrook, NJ 08302-0655, (609) 455-7575, Edward M. Diehl, President

Seniors Management, Inc. 1114 Wynwood Avenue, Cherry Hill, NJ 08002, (609) 663-4044, Robert J. Sall, President

Shoreline Behavioral Health Center, Inc. *(Founded 1987)* 1691 Route 9, Toms River, NJ 08755, (908) 914-1688, Kenneth E. Bonaly, President and CEO

Shore Memorial Hospital *(Founded 1928)* New York Avenue, Somers Point, NJ 08244, (609) 653-3500, Richard A. Pitman, President

Somerset Medical Center *(Founded 1901)* 110 Rehill Avenue, Somerville, NJ 08876, (908) 685-2200, William J. Monagle, FACHE, President and CEO

South Amboy Memorial Hospital *(Founded 1918)* 540 Bordentown Avenue, South Amboy, NJ 08879, (908) 721-1000, Irv J. Diamond, Chief Executive Officer

Southern Ocean County Hospital *(Founded 1972)* 1140 West Bay Avenue, Route 72, Manahawkin, NJ 08050, (609) 597-6011, Steven G. Littleson, President and CEO

South Jersey Hospital System 333 Irving Avenue, Bridgeton, NJ 08302-2100, (609) 451-6600, Paul S. Cooper, President and CEO

    Bridgeton Division *(Founded 1898)* 333 Irving Avenue, Bridgeton, NJ 08302-2100, (609) 451-6600

    Millville Division *(Founded 1915)* 1200 N. High Street, Millville, NJ 08332-2586, (609) 825-3500

Sunrise House Foundation, Inc. *(Founded 1983)* Sunset Inn Road, P.O. Box 600, Lafayette, NJ 07848, (201) 383-6300, Beth Ann Nathans, Chief Executive Officer

T

Trenton Psychiatric Hospital *(Founded 1848)* Route 29 and Sullivan Way, P.O. Box 7500, West Trenton, NJ 08628, (609) 633-1500, Joseph Jupin, Jr., Acting CEO

U

Underwood–Memorial Hospital *(Founded 1907)* 509 N. Broad Street, P.O. Box 359, Woodbury, NJ 08096-7358, (609) 845-0100, William D. Thompson, President

Union Hospital *(Founded 1944)* 1000 Galloping Hill Road, Union, NJ 07083, (908) 687-1900, Victor J. Fresolone, FACHE, FCOHE, President and CEO

United Hospitals Medical Center *(Founded 1959)* 15 South Ninth Street, Newark, NJ 07107, (201) 268-8000, John Dandridge, Jr., President and CEO

University of Medicine and Dentistry of New Jersey–University Hospital *(Founded 1882)* 150 Bergen Street, Newark, NJ 07103-2425, (201) 982-4300, Marc H. Lory, Vice President and CEO

The Valley Hospital *(Founded 1951)* 223 North Van Dien Avenue, Ridgewood, NJ 07450, (201) 447-8000, Michael W. Azzara, President

V

Veterans Affairs Medical Center *(Founded 1952)* Tremont Avenue & S. Centre Street, East Orange, NJ 07019, (201) 676-1000, Kenneth H. Mizrach, Director

Veterans Affairs Medical Center *(Founded 1930)* Lyons, NJ 07939, (908) 647-0180, A. Paul Kidd, FACHE, Medical Center Director

W

Wallkill Valley Hospital and Health Centers *(Founded 1908)* 20 Walnut Street, Sussex, NJ 07461, (201) 702-2200, John J. Farley, Chief Executive Officer

Warren Hospital *(Founded 1921)* 185 Roseberry Street, Phillipsburg, NJ 08865, (908) 859-6700, John A. DeMarrais, President

Wayne General Hospital *(Founded 1871)* 224 Hamburg Turnpike, Wayne, NJ 07470, (201) 956-3500, Justin E. Doheny, President and CEO

Welkind Rehabilitation Hospital *(Founded 1962)* (Formerly Multiple Sclerosis Service Organization of New Jersey) Pleasant Hill Road, Chester, NJ 07930, (201) 584-7500, Kenneth W. Aitchison, President and CEO

Well Care Group, Inc. 250 Old Hook Road, Westwood, NJ 07675, (201) 358-3014, Louis R. Ycre, Jr., President

    Pascack Valley Hospital *(Founded 1959)* Old Hook Road, Westwood, NJ 07675, (201) 358-3000

West Hudson Hospital *(Founded 1913)* 206 Bergen Avenue, Kearny, NJ 07032, (201) 955-7000, Carmen B. Alecci, Chief Executive Officer

West Jersey Health System Corporate Office, 1000 Atlantic Avenue, Camden, NJ 08104, (609) 342-4000, Barry D. Brown, President and CEO

    West Jersey Hospital–Berlin *(Founded 1965)* (Formerly Southern Division) White Horse Pike & Townsend Avenue, Berlin, NJ 08009, (609) 768-6006

    West Jersey Hospital–Camden *(Founded 1885)* (Formerly Northern Division) 1000 Atlantic Avenue, Camden, NJ 08104, (609) 342-4572

    West Jersey Hospital–Marlton *(Founded 1973)* (Formerly Garden State Community Hospital) Route 73 & Brick Road, Marlton, NJ 08053, (609) 596-3700

    West Jersey Hospital–Voorhees *(Founded 1973)* (Formerly Eastern Division) 101 Carnie Blvd., Voorhees, NJ 08043, (609) 772-5500

William B. Kessler Memorial Hospital *(Founded 1963)* 600 South White Horse Pike, Hammonton, NJ 08037-2099, (609) 561-6700, Warren E. Gager, Chief Executive Officer

Z

Zurbrugg Memorial Hospital (See **Graduate Health System, Inc.**)

ALLIED ORGANIZATIONS*

A

Association of Family Practice Nurse Managers (609) 795-4330, (908)545-6303, Ex. 205, Jeannette Eckert, R.N., President

Association of Healthcare Executives of New Jersey (201) 795-7017, Bernadette Norz, President

Association of Institutional Linen Managers (201) 285-2851, Leon Presciepa, President

Association for Practitioners in Infection Control North New Jersey (201) 441-2064, Nancy Nelsen, R.N., B.S., CIC, President; South New Jersey (908) 828-3000, Arlene Potts, MPHCIC, President

C

Council of Hospital Physical Therapy Directors (908) 668-2195, Alice Kiemle, President

DRG Management Association (201) 625-1655, Alma Ratcliffe, President

Executive Hospital Engineers of New Jersey, Inc. (201) 989-3177, Charles F. Church, Chief Engineer

Greater New Jersey Society for Hospital Food Service Administrators (201) 451-9000, Garry Feverberg, President

H

Healthcare Data Processing Management Association (609) 275-4216, Richard D. Weaver, President

Health Care Executive Forum (609) 825-3500, Ronald P. Sotak, President

Healthcare Financial Management Association of New Jersey (201) 894-3280, Douglas A. Duchak, President

Health Care Materials Management Society of New Jersey, Inc. (609) 936-2195, Phyllis Molnar Tutek, President

Healthcare Planning and Marketing Society of New Jersey (609) 394-4254, Andrea Miller, President

Healthcare Quality Professionals of New Jersey (908) 937-8618, Judith Evans, President

Health Sciences Library Association of New Jersey (201) 996-2326, Duressa Pujat, President

Hospital Engineers Association of Southern New Jersey (609) 582-2546, James A. Weikel, President

Hospital Fund Raising Executives of New Jersey (HFRENJ) (908) 530-2490, John Nolan, President

National Executive Housekeepers Association, Inc., Garden State Chapter (201) 831-5095, Gregory M. Ogden, REH, President

New Jersey Association of Directors of Volunteer Services (908) 499-6037, Phyllis Andelman, President

N

New Jersey Association of Health Care Access Management (908) 522-2078, Sondra Rizkalla, A.A.M., President

New Jersey Association of Hospital Recruiters (609) 599-5619, Rita Bell, President

New Jersey Association of Mobile Intensive Care Unit Program Administration (609) 394-6064, Robert Hartman, President

New Jersey Chapter of the Society of Patient Representation – Consumer Affairs AHA (908) 321-7902, Caryl A. Distel, President

New Jersey Chapter, The College of Chaplains (908) 530-8236, Rev. Joseph Nilsen, President

New Jersey Dietetic Association (201) 456-6731, Geri McKay, M.Ed. RD, President

New Jersey Healthcare Central Service Association (908) 780-6085, Jacqueline McCullough, President

New Jersey Healthcare Media Association (609) 394-6000, Joseph T. Zalescik, President

New Jersey Health Care Public Relations and Marketing Association (201) 977-2043, Rita Rooney, President

New Jersey Hospital Employee Health Nurses Association (609) 394-6278, Joan Donigan, President

New Jersey Hospital Security and Safety Directors Association (908) 823-3000, Douglas Campbell, President

New Jersey Hospital Telecommunications Association (201) 967-4299/4000, Don Cumming, President

New Jersey Information Management Association (609) 936-2223, Colleen Donnelly, Director

New Jersey Patient Account Managers Association, Inc. (201) 977-2301, Denis Hemingway, President

New Jersey Patient Transport Association (NJPTA) (609) 599-5000, Connie Wilson, L.P.N., President

New Jersey Society, American Association of Respiratory Care (201) 625-6723, Sharon Williams Colon, President

New Jersey Society for Clinical Laboratory Management (908) 295-6444, Elosie R. Eith, President

New Jersey Society for Healthcare Education and Training (SHET/NJ) (908) 776-4132, Bernice L. Scott, President

New Jersey Society for Healthcare Human Resources Administrators (201) 625-6000, Jacalyn Bidwell, Vice President

New Jersey Society for Medical Technology (201) 457-6863, Nadine Fydryszewski

New Jersey Society of Hospital Pharmacists (908) 522-2222, Jeannie Cirillo, President

New Jersey Society of Hospital Social Work Directors (908) 851-7049, Victoria Hasser, President

New York/New Jersey Association for Healthcare Philanthropy (AHP), Region III (201) 447-8089, Allen J. O'Keefe, President

S

Senior Health Care Executive Society of New Jersey (201) 625-6000, Stan Sebastian, President

Society for Health Care Risk Management of New Jersey (201) 533-8259, Karen G. Seiden, President

*as of 12/31/92

ACKNOWLEDGMENTS
The authors would like to especially thank the following people at the New Jersey Hospital Association for their assistance in researching this book: Diana Stager, Vice President, Planning; Ron Czajkowski, Vice President, Communications; Keri Ellerbroek, Director of Publications; Michelle Volesko, Director of Library and Corporate Information Services for the J. Harold Johnston Memorial Library at the Health Research and Educational Trust of New Jersey; and Angela Harris-Scriven, Library Research Associate.

The New Jersey Hospital Association *75th Anniversary*
CELEBRATING INNOVATIVE LEADERSHIP IN HEALTHCARE
By Virginia Persing, Trish Krotowski

Edited by Nancy Jackson
Senior Editor, Jeffrey Reeves
Contributing Writer, Rod Hirsch

Designed by Tom Lewis, Inc.
Photo Editor, Robin L. Sterling

Managing Editor: Linda J. Hreno. *Coordinator:* Kelly Goulding. *Proofreaders:* Martha Cheresh, Lin Schonberger. *Editorial Assistant:* Kimberly J. Pelletier. *Assistant Coordinators:* Keith Martin, Erin Goulding.

Production Manager: Jeffrey Scott Hayes. *Art Production:* Amanda J. Howard. *Manager, Computer Systems:* Steve Zehngut. *Art Production Consulting:* Jonathan Wieder.

Marketing: Nancy Freidin, Claire Paul-Cook. *Book Orders:* Connie Black. *Account Manager:* Carolyn Martin. *Accounting:* Linda Reeves. *Office Services:* Kimberly Larson, Michael Nugwynne, Carolyn Kenney.

Published in cooperation with the New Jersey Hospital Association by Windsor Publications, Inc., 21827 Nordhoff Street, Chatsworth, CA 91311. Elliot Martin, *Chairman of the Board and CEO.* J. Kelley Younger, *Publisher and Editor-in-Chief.* Terry Pender, *Controller* .

Produced with the support of CCA Publications, Inc., Nellie Scott, *President.*

Library of Congress Cataloging-in-Publication Data

Persing, Virginia
    Celebrating innovative leadership in healthcare / Virginia Persing, Trish Krotowski.
    p.144 cm. 25 x 31
    At head of title: The New Jersey Hospital Association 75th Anniversary.
    "Partners in progress," Rod Hirsch.
    ISBN 0-89781-470-3 : $34.95
    1. Hospitals—New Jersey—History. 2. Hospital Care—New Jersey—History. 3. New Jersey Hospital Association—History.
I. Krotowski, Trish. II. Hirsch, Rod. III. New Jersey Hospital Association. IV. Title.
    [DNLM: 1. New Jersey Hospital Association. 2. Delivery of Health Care—history—New Jersey. 3. Hospitals—history—New Jersey. WX 11 AN4 P4c 1993]
RA981.N5P47 1993
362.1'1'09749—dc20
DNLM/DLC
for Library of Congress   93-3473